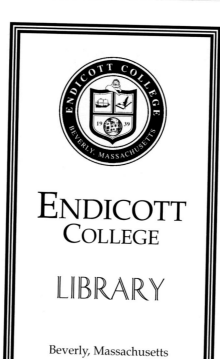

ENDICOTT
COLLEGE

LIBRARY

Beverly, Massachusetts

PANOS DOSSIER

AIDS AND THE THIRD WORLD

published in association with
the Norwegian Red Cross

The Panos Institute

London — Paris — Washington

New Society Publishers

Philadelphia, PA — Santa Cruz, CA

Non-trade editions published 1986, 1987
Trade edition 1989

Inquiries regarding requests to reprint all or part of this book should be addressed to:
New Society Publishers
4527 Springfield Avenue
Philadelphia, PA 19143, USA.

ISBN 0-86571-143-7 Hardcover
ISBN 0-86571-144-5 Paperback

Production: Jacqueline Walkden and Gillian Hitchcock.
Picture research: Patricia Lee.
Cover design: Robert Purnell.
Maps and graphs: Philip Davies.
Printed in the USA on partially recycled paper by R.R. Donnelley and Sons.

The work of the Panos AIDS Unit is supported financially by the Norwegian Red
Cross and the Norwegian Ministry for Development Cooperation.

Any judgements expressed in this document should not be taken to represent the
views of any funding agency.

This dossier was written by Renée Sabatier, with contributions from Martin
Foreman, who also compiled Appendix One and Two. It was edited by Jon
Tinker. Marty Radlett contributed additional research and writing in Chapter
Eight, and Tisa Hughes provided additional research throughout. Elizabeth Cecil
compiled source material for Chapter Two. Patricia Ardila of Panos Washington
helped with US source material.

The Panos Institute is an international information and policy studies institute,
dedicated to working in partnership with others towards greater public
understanding of sustainable development. Panos has offices in Washington DC,
London and Paris and was founded in 1986 by the staff of Earthscan, which has
undertaken similar work since 1975.

For more information about Panos contact:
The Panos Institute, 1409 King Street
Alexandria, VA 22314, USA.

To order books directly from the publisher, please add US$1.75 shipping and
handling for the first copy, US$0.50 each additional copy. Send your check or
money order to New Society Publishers/West, PO Box 582, Santa Cruz, CA
95061, USA.

New Society Publishers is a project of the New Society Educational Foundation,
a nonprofit, tax-exempt, public foundation. Opinions expressed in this book do
not necessarily represent positions of the New Society Educational Foundation.

AIDS: THE CHANGING PICTURE

THE interlinked health, development and humanitarian crises caused by AIDS have become steadily more severe since the first edition of *AIDS and the Third World* was published in November 1986.

True, the present extent and possible future impacts of the emerging AIDS pandemic have sometimes been exaggerated. But it is becoming more and more clear that estimates from the World Health Organization and from national health authorities have in fact usually been *under*stated. As figures and graphs throughout this dossier indicate, new AIDS cases continue to rise more steeply, and only among homosexual men in the United States and a few European countries are there signs of a slowdown in the growth of HIV infection.

Worldwide, it seems likely that a new person becomes infected with the HIV virus every minute. During 1988, 150,000 new cases of full-blown AIDS are expected — as many as are thought to have ocurred in all the years of the epidemic so far.

The global spread

The first major change in the AIDS situation since late 1986 has been the insidious entry of HIV to virtually every corner of the globe (see Appendix I). Then, the first edition of this dossier concentrated heavily on Africa, because little data was available from other parts of the Third World. This third edition is much more truly global. While AIDS is only starting to gain a foothold in Asia, the Middle East and East Europe, there are now epidemics in Latin America and the Caribbean as severe as — and in many cases more severe than — those in North America, West Europe and Australasia. Previous claims that religion, culture or ideology afford effective protection from the AIDS virus have proved unfounded.

In Africa, AIDS has from its inception been transmitted heterosexually, rather than homosexually as was at first almost entirely the case in North America and Europe. Now, in the Americas outside the USA and Canada, a disquieting pattern is emerging. As Chapter Three describes, the evidence clearly suggests that the heterosexual transmission of HIV is steadily taking hold, particularly in parts of the Caribbean and Central America. And as women in their child-bearing years become infected with HIV, more societies are having to grapple with the medical and human tragedies of babies born with the virus, most *'like a misery-seeking missile'*

of whom will die before their second birthday. Panos has just started a study on AIDS as a disease of the family, and on the ways that it affect children and their mothers. We hope to publish a report in mid-1989.

Governments take action

The unrelieved bleakness of this picture has been lightened by a second major change since 1986: in global terms governments and the international system have responded to the challenge of AIDS with a speed and vigour that is probably unprecedented. The first edition of this dossier commented forcefully on the failure of governments to take AIDS seriously; today, governmental recognition is widespread. By mid-1988, 176 of the world's countries had joined WHO's global AIDS reporting network; 138 had reported cases of AIDS, and 151 had established national AIDS committees.

Relatively few heads of government have yet personally committed themselves to these anti-AIDS mobilisations, with the notable exceptions of two African presidents: Yoweri Museveni of Uganda, and Kenneth Kaunda of Zambia. These two leaders have played a key role in persuading decisionmakers and media in some other African countries to abandon their earlier reticence in discussing AIDS, and in making AIDS statistics available.

Yet the potential long-term effects of AIDS are still little appreciated. Mathematical models of AIDS epidemiology, based on conservative estimates of present infection, suggest that AIDS in some African countries is likely to reverse population growth over a period of decades, unless current trends in infection and mortality can be changed. These same models, as Chapter Four discusses, indicate that once heterosexual transmission becomes a real factor, AIDS has a destructive potential greater than that of bubonic plague. The difference is that the impact of AIDS will take much longer to show up: decades instead of years.

In this respect AIDS is an even *more* dangerous threat than plague, because it operates on so much longer a timescale. Nearly all governments are finding it hard to handle an epidemic whose impacts will mount for decades, and where essential countermeasures will not show any obvious benefits for five or ten years.

A third major change since the first issue of this dossier has been the emergence of AIDS as (another) disease of disadvantage and deprivation. This has been delineated most sharply in the United States, perhaps because that country now records and analyses its statistics in racial, ethnic and geographical terms, but the same pattern is visible, if less clearly, in many other nations, as well as on the international scale.

The picture that is taking shape is of a virus which behaves like a misery-seeking missile, seeking out populations made doubly vulnerable by their lack of information, and by their health, behavioural and socio-economic status. As Chapter Four describes, both within the United States, and globally as between countries and continents, AIDS is more and more becoming a disease that hits people of colour. The long-term political effects this may bring should not be underestimated.

Scientific developments

A fourth change since 1986 has been a new chapter in the vexed search for the origins of AIDS, and of the virus that causes it. The most recent research (see Chapter Three of this dossier) has made untenable the controversial hypothesis that the AIDS virus jumped from African green monkeys to African people in recent years. Those wild monkeys do carry *a* virus, but the indications are that this virus is not the parent of the human AIDS viruses, whose origins remain as obscure as ever.

A fifth significant development has been three shifts of emphasis on the scientific front, which are discussed in Chapter Two. In 1986, most health authorities were insisting in public that there was no good evidence that more than 10-30% of those infected by the HIV virus would eventually develop AIDS. In the first edition of this dossier, The Panos Institute warned that in private many virologists considered it probable that the death rate from HIV infection would eventually climb towards 100%. Panos was criticised for this reporting in 1986; by mid-1988, the medical consensus had substantially altered. It is now recognised that few of those infected with HIV escape harmful effects; and the appearance of harmful effects is increasingly recognised as a prelude to eventual AIDS.

The second shift in scientific opinion has been the sober realisation that, barring an unexpected scientific breakthrough, the development of a vaccine to give effective protection against HIV infection is unlikely in the forseeable future. In 1986, the scientific consensus was that with luck a vaccine might be available by 1995; today, that prospect looks distinctly optimistic.

The third shift in medical views has been more hopeful. In 1986, the tendency was to assume that once a person had developed clear symptoms of AIDS, death would almost always follow within a couple of years. In the last two years, an increasing number of PWAs (people with AIDS) in Europe and North America have been able, with the use of drugs such as AZT, with careful diet and lifestyle, and with a positive personal attitide combined with support from family and friends, to live full and rewarding lives for far longer than was previously thought possible.

Many PWAs are now playing a key role in fighting the epidemic. At a recent Panos seminar, two speakers were PWAs; between them, they had lived 13 years since being diagnosed with AIDS.

'a tendency to blame others'

A fifth major development has been the universality of the social tendency to deny that AIDS is affecting our own communities. This has delayed, and continues to delay, our response to the challenge of HIV.

Denial and blame

Denial has in nearly every country been followed by a tendency to blame others for introducing and for spreading HIV. The United States has blamed homosexual men and Haitians; Europeans and Indians have blamed Africans; Africans have blamed Europeans; Asians have blamed American seamen; others have blamed students, or foreigners, or prostitutes, or ethnic minorities, or capitalists, or unbelievers. These epidemics of blame and counter-blame are described in Chapter Six, and are documented more fully in the 1988 Panos book *Blaming Others: Prejudice, race and worldwide AIDS*, by Renée Sabatier and 12 Third World co-authors (see inside back cover).

As denial has been followed by blame, so blame has often been followed by stigmatisation, by discrimination, and by persecution: directed against people with AIDS, against those who are HIV-positive, or against individuals or groups perceived as being likely to be infected: see Chapter Nine.

The World Health Organization has repeatedly challenged this tendency. Said Dr Jonathan Mann, head of WHO's AIDS programme, to the Stockholm AIDS conference in June 1988: "In thinking about AIDS some seek to oppose the 'right of the many' to remain uninfected against the 'rights of the few' who are already HIV infected. This is a false dilemma, for the protection of the uninfected majority depends precisely upon and is inextricably bound with the protection of the rights and dignity of infected persons". The chairman of the US Presidential AIDS Commission made the same point in the same month: "HIV-related discrimination is impairing this nation's ability to limit the spread of the epidemic". In collaboration with the Norwegian Red Cross and WHO, Panos has started an investigation of these and other humanitarian aspects of AIDS.

A start on education

The sixth significant change in the AIDS scene since 1986 has been that AIDS education has begun in earnest in scores of countries. It is too early yet to say whether it is working, in terms of persuading people to change their sexual behaviour so as to reduce their exposure to HIV. But as Chapter Five of this dossier shows, there are many hopeful signs. More and more communities are beginning to mobilise, to educate and to protect themselves. The challenge for governments is not simply to carry out such education, but to foster the political, social and legal environments which contribute to the open and effective communication of AIDS information.

AIDS is a fast-changing field. As a result, this dossier has been about 80% rewritten since its second edition in March 1987. Panos does not anticipate publishing a fourth edition, since it is becoming increasingly difficult to document developments in a book before they have become out of date.

Instead, The Panos Institute hopes by late 1988 to start publication, in collaboration with the London Bureau of Hygiene and Tropical Diseases and other partners, of a regular newsletter called *WorldAIDS*. It will have the same emphases as this dossier: a comprehensive global overview of AIDS, an inter-disciplinary content, and an emphasis on AIDS as it affects the Third World.

Jon Tinker
President
The Panos Institute

CONTENTS

Hundreds of individuals and organisations supplied information for this dossier. Space unfortunately prevents naming them, but Panos is immensely grateful for their assistance. Special thanks are due to those PWAs (people with AIDS) who so generously spent time explaining and commenting on parts of the material contained in the text.

In particular Panos would like to thank its AIDS Advisory Panel, whose advice, criticism and support has made this and other AIDS Unit publications possible. Members of the panel have read and commented on all or part of the manuscript of this dossier, and in most cases their suggestions have been incorporated. The responsibility for any errors or omissions, however, rests with Panos, and the text should not be taken to represent the exact views of all the panel members.

ADVISORY PANEL

Calle Almedal, Nordic Red Cross AIDS Coordinator, Norwegian Red Cross, Oslo, Norway.
Dr Johnathan Mann, Director, Global Programme on AIDS, WHO, Geneva, Switzerland.
Dr Jean William Pape, Assistant Professor of Medicine, Cornell University Medical College and State University of Haiti (Port au Prince).
Dr Anthony Pinching, Consultant Immunologist, St Mary's Hospital, London, UK.
Dr Peter Piot, Head, Department of Microbiology, Institute of Tropical Medicine, Antwerp, Belgium.
Dr Pramilla Senanayake, Assistant Secretary General, technical services, Interational Planned Parenthood Federation, London, UK.
Dr Richard Tedder, Head, Department of Virology, Middlesex Hospital Medical School, London, UK.

CHAPTER ONE

WHAT IS AIDS?

AIDS is a disease* caused by a new and deadly virus: *HIV* (the Human Immunodeficiency Virus). HIV can remain in the body for years, perhaps even decades, before any damage shows up as visible symptoms. Once AIDS develops, in all known cases it has always proved fatal. At present, there is no cure for AIDS, and no vaccine is available to protect against it.

The term *AIDS* (Acquired Immune Deficiency Syndrome) refers, strictly speaking, only to the last, fatal stage of HIV infection, which is often also called *"full-blown AIDS"*.

In non-medical literature the term AIDS is also used, rather more loosely, to refer to earlier stages of HIV infection, and to the virus epidemic which by the end of June 1988 had reached at least 138 of the 176 countries and territories now reporting on AIDS to the World Health Organization (WHO). Such a widespread epidemic is called a *pandemic*.

For the virus which causes AIDS, the internationally accepted name is now HIV. The HIV virus was previously called *HTLV-3* (the US name) and *LAV* (the French name); these terms are used now less and less often in medical journals and the media.

In general usage, the terms HIV, the AIDS virus, HTLV-3 and LAV now mean the same thing. This chapter looks at the AIDS virus which was discovered first and which is more widespread HIV-1; the second AIDS virus, HIV-2, and other variants, are discussed in Chapter Three.

HIV and its target cells

Viruses are the smallest of all disease-producing organisms: much smaller than bacteria, and far too small to be visible through an ordinary microscope. Influenza, polio, the common cold and smallpox are just a few of the illnesses caused by viruses.

A virus can only reproduce within the living cell of a larger

---

The term "disease" is used in this document as a shorthand way of referring to AIDS. In reality AIDS is, strictly speaking, not a disease but a collection of 70 or more conditions which result from the damage done to the immune system and other parts of the body as a result of infection by the AIDS virus. AIDS is thus more accurately referred to as a "syndrome" — a collection of various symptoms, infections and conditions.

Figure 1.1
This T4 helper cell is
infected with HIV.
The virus is
multiplying rapidly
within the cell and is
"budding" on its
surface, ready to
burst out of the cell,
killing it and going
on to infect other
lymphocytes.
[Magnification:
20,000X]

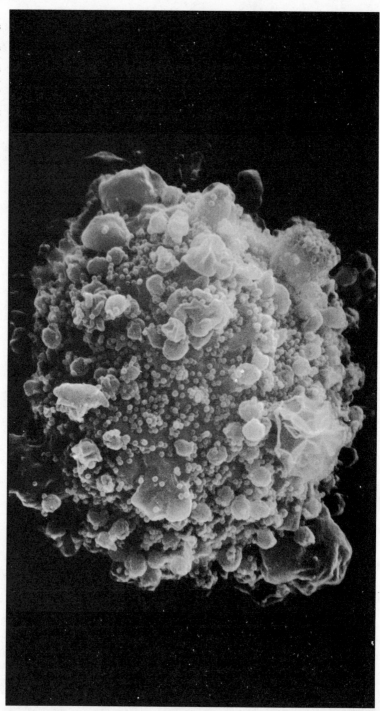

NIBSC

organism. Once inside, the virus may kill the host cell, alter its functioning, or simply "sleep": remaining hidden within the host cell, more or less inactive, sometimes for a very long time.

The human body is equipped with a large number of white blood cells, which mount a two-tiered defence against invaders like viruses. The first line of defence is made up of *scavenger cells*, and the second line is *lymphocytes*; both are types of white blood cells. Scavenger cells are manufactured in the bone marrow and found in most body tissues. Scavengers are present to recognise, engulf and "eat" invaders, other foreign material and cell debris. HIV can infect a type of long-lived scavenger cell called *macrophages*, and may pass from them to infect certain other body cells [1].

'the ability to resist infections is progressively diminished'

Macrophage scavengers are the body's first defence against an invading disease organism: they can call for reinforcements by signalling lymphocytes. Together, the scavenger cells and the lymphocytes constitute the major part of the body's *immune system*, the proper functioning of which allows us to live in a world where there are millions of potentially deadly infective viruses and bacteria.

Lymphocytes are the prime movers in the body's immune response to disease organisms. They constitute a highly specialised team of defenders, patrolling the blood and body looking for intruders such as viruses. Circulating lymphocytes are mainly the *T-cells*, which can recognise the precise biochemical identity of an invader. When they find an invader, T-cells instruct a second part of the lymphocyte team, the *B-cells*, to produce precision proteins called antibodies. These neutralise the virus by attaching to it, each antibody recognising only one specific virus.

T-lymphocytes, in addition to helping B-cells make antibodies, have other functions critical for our resistance to disease. A T-cell sub-group, the *T4 helper cells,* plays a key co-ordinating role in the body's immune response to the threat of infection. Unique among known viruses, HIV can insert itself into these helper cells, and over a period of months or years destroy them. When this happens, communication within the immune system goes awry, and the person's ability to resist all manner of infections is progressively diminished.

The T-helper cells act as "mission control" within the immune system. For example, they regulate the activity of yet another T-cell sub-group, the *killer T-cells*. Killer cells are specialised assassins, and left to themselves they might not only kill infected cells, but also healthy cells vital to the body's functioning. To do their job these killers must be able to distinguish between infected and uninfected cells. And when their job is finished — when the virus is defeated — the body's supply of killer cells must be damped down. T4 helper cells are instrumental in co-ordinating both these tasks.

'*anti-HIV antibodies do not appear to neutralise the virus*'

There is much that is still unknown about the way in which the AIDS virus gets into T-helper cells. HIV may enter the bloodstream and infect helper cells directly [2]. Alternatively, it may first infect the scavenging macrophage cells, which could then pass the virus to the helper cells [3]. And recently it has been shown that HIV can possibly infect still another type of body cell, the *Langerhans* cells which are present in mucous membranes lining the mouth, lungs, genital and anal regions and the cornea of the eye [4]. These cells, too, might act as a reservoir of HIV, allowing for the eventual infection of the T-helper cells.

Whatever the sequence of events that leads to T-helper cell infection, AIDS is the devastating end result. HIV replicates within the infected helper cells, killing them as it bursts out to colonise still more of them. It is not yet clear what triggers these destructive bursts of viral replication. One unpleasant theory is that the dormant AIDS virus becomes active and multiplies when the body is responding to a new disease threat. The biochemical signal which stimulates T-cells to divide and activate the rest of the immune system may instead trigger the AIDS virus to replicate, destroying in the process the very T-helper cells which co-ordinate the immune response [5].

The ineffectiveness of antibodies to HIV

Why is it, researchers would like to know, that the antibodies to HIV produced by the B-lymphocytes seem to be ineffective against the virus? Normally, after an antibody has stopped a particular virus from multiplying, the B-cells stop producing that antibody. But they remember how to produce it, should the invader return. Antibodies and the cells producing them are the human body's "memory" of past invaders; the presence of a particular antibody in the blood shows that the virus was once there. This memory makes a powerful, often impregnable, defence against any new attack by the same virus.

The lymphocyte defence team of co-ordinated T and B cells can take a while to identify the invading virus and then to produce enough antibodies to overwhelm it. Meanwhile, the virus may be multiplying in the body, altering the chemistry of its cells, and making the person ill. If the lymphocytes work fast enough, their antibodies eventually overwhelm the virus. The presence of antibodies in the blood is normally a healthy sign: it means that the lymphocytes are responding to the viral attack. If they do not, the invading virus may be able to kill or badly damage its victim.

Though infection by HIV is usually followed by the production of anti-HIV antibodies, these do not appear to neutralise the virus. This may be because HIV, for much of the time it is present in the body, successfully hides from antibodies inside the T-cells, macrophages or other cells it infects [6]. But it seems that too few T-cells are actually infected by HIV to account for the tremendous damage it does to the immune system [7]. Some virologists think that, from within the T-cells it infects, HIV may secrete proteins that stick to numbers of healthy T-cells. Deceived by these sticky viral proteins, anti-HIV antibodies may then also clump onto these T-cells, which are eventually destroyed in the process [8].

'eventually the person with AIDS will die'

Though they do not succeed in eliminating HIV from the body, HIV antibodies (which are antibodies produced against HIV and which immunologists call "anti-HIV antibodies") can be detected in blood tests. Since detecting the virus itself is extremely difficult, testing for antibodies to HIV is now the standard way of finding out if a person is a HIV-carrier. If such a test shows that HIV antibodies are present in the blood, the person is said to be *HIV-positive* or *seropositive*.

A HIV-positive blood test does not mean someone has AIDS. It is therefore *not* an "AIDS test", though it is often mistakenly referred to in this way. It does mean he or she has antibodies to HIV. Since we know that the virus is not destroyed by these antibodies, virologists assume that anyone with antibodies to HIV is at risk of eventually developing AIDS (see Chapter Two).

AIDS: the disease

The AIDS virus gradually disables the body's immune system. The infected person becomes increasingly vulnerable to almost any infection — by another virus, a bacterium, a fungus or a parasite. These *opportunistic* infections mainly occur in the skin, the lungs, the digestive system, the nervous system and the brain. He or she suffers a long period of illness and disease. Medical treatment — for pneumonia, for example — may for a time make the symptoms less unpleasant. But eventually the person with AIDS will die, usually within two or three years of diagnosis.

It seems likely that a number of "co-factors" — other infections, the use of drugs, sexual behaviour (including multiple partners), and possibly also pregnancy — may accelerate the HIV infection from one stage to the next, possibly by stimulating the virus to replicate and infect more cells.

In theory (but not always in practice), there are five stages in the development of HIV infection. Both WHO and the US Centers for Disease Control (CDC) have produced a "case definition" of AIDS. These are sets of guidelines outlining symptoms and signs which physicians can use when attempting to diagnose AIDS. (The CDC case definition was expanded in 1987 to include symptoms of dementia and prolonged weight loss.) The five stages are:

- initial HIV infection
- PGL: persistently enlarged lymph glands
- ARC: AIDS-related complex
- full-blown AIDS
- AIDS dementia

Not every infected person goes through each stage. Some patients show no obvious signs of illness before developing full-blown AIDS. Others may live for months or even years with no symptoms beyond enlarged glands in the neck.

Recently the US National Academy of Sciences, in its second authoritative report on AIDS, stated its view that the terms PGL and ARC are no longer scientifically useful because they do not help physicians to predict whether or not an HIV-infected patient will go on to develop AIDS. The stage to which the seropositive individual's infection has progressed is more accurately described by a combination of symptoms and laboratory tests assessing immune dysfunction, the report says [9]. The terms PGL and ARC are used in this dossier because they help the layperson to visualise the kinds of symptoms associated with HIV infection and AIDS.

The typical symptoms of each of the five stages are summarised below. This is based largely on North American and European experience; the syndrome varies considerably from one part of the world to another, and less clinical research is available on AIDS patients in developing countries.

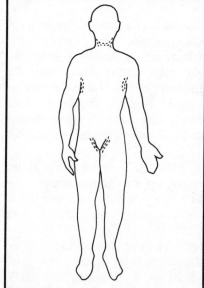

Figure 1.2 Persistently enlarged lymph glands, in the neck, armpit or groin are one of the early symptoms which can signal infection by the HIV virus.

Initial HIV infection: Within a few weeks of HIV entering the body, some people experience a temporary "seroconversion illness", which may resemble influenza or glandular fever (infectious mononucleosis). During this time the immune system produces antibodies to HIV which do not succeed in overcoming the virus. This is usually followed by a period of months or years in which no further symptoms appear, but during which the person is capable of transmitting the virus to others.

PGL (which stands for persistent generalised lymphadenopathy): Enlarged lymph glands, in the neck, armpit or groin can follow this initial bout of illness and may be accompanied by fevers, night sweats, loss of weight and oral thrush (a fungus infection inside the mouth). For many people in developed countries, these symptoms are often the first which prompt a visit to the doctor. But for many people living in Third World conditions, such symptoms may be all but indistinguishable from common infections for which treatment is either unavailable or rarely sought.

ARC (which stands for AIDS-related complex): The AIDS virus has by now damaged the immune system considerably. Many opportunistic infections occur. Symptoms include fatigue, unexplained diarrhoea lasting longer than one month, loss of more than 10% of body weight, fevers and night sweats. Oral thrush, PGL, or enlarged spleen may be present.

Full-blown AIDS: The immune system is collapsing. Major life-threatening infections invade the body. These vary among patients and among countries. Pneumonia caused by the parasitic *Pneumocystis carinii* is common in the United States, as is a cancer affecting the skin called Kaposi's sarcoma. In parts of Africa a wasting condition called "slim disease", linked to persistent diarrhoea, is common. The AIDS patient is usually extremely thin and grossly fatigued, and has multiple infections such as shingles, thrush, herpes and tuberculosis. Full-blown AIDS seems to be always fatal: few people diagnosed with it have lived longer than three to four years.

AIDS dementia (or AIDS dementia complex): The AIDS virus can pass through the blood-brain barrier, which normally "filters out" substances in the blood which might damage the brain. Once past this barrier, HIV can destroy certain brain cells, causing symptoms ranging from mild confusion, memory loss, deteriorating thought processes and inappropriate behaviour to personality change, premature senility and incontinence. The normally young victim may require complete care for as long as he or she lives. The majority of AIDS patients develop some signs of brain or nervous system involvement, and there have been reports of patients who developed neurological symptoms in advance of developing full-blown AIDS [10]. But an international group of experts assembled by WHO found no evidence that people infected with the AIDS virus were likely to suffer significant mental disturbances before exhibiting the disease itself [11].

Testing for antibodies

The body defends itself against each new virus infection by manufacturing precision-tailored proteins called antibodies, whose presence indicates prior exposure to infection. As we age we thus become walking antibody "catalogues" of the infections we have come into contact with. It is thought that nearly everyone who has been exposed to HIV produces antibodies against it.

To detect these HIV antibodies in the blood, a number of different tests have been developed, notably in the United States, United Kingdom, France and the Netherlands. First invented in 1983, the tests became commercially available in 1984. None of them is infallible. Two of the currently most widely used tests are known as the ELISA and the Western Blot.

People infected by HIV do not produce antibodies for an average period of six weeks to three months. The virus is present in their blood, but the blood tests cannot detect it because they are designed to register the presence of HIV antibodies rather than HIV itself. Blood tests carried out on recently infected people can therefore give *false-negative* results, though improvements in the technology of testing are narrowing the time "window" during which such false results can occur. A small minority of people appear never to produce antibodies against HIV, even though the virus itself is hiding in their bodies.

Scientific reports also indicate that, probably infrequently, individuals who have tested positive for HIV antibodies appear, on later retesting, to have lost these antibodies [12]. Testing for the virus itself is possible, but it is expensive, cumbersome and not yet commercially practical. However, very recently a new method of registering the presence of HIV in blood samples, called the *polymerase chain reaction*, has been developed. This test may soon become widely available, and it has already given rise to disquieting evidence that in some cases people who are carrying the virus may not produce any antibodies to it — and thus appear seronegative when given the standard anti-HIV antibody blood test [13].

Blood tests can also give *false-positive* results: they may indicate that a person has been exposed to the virus when in fact he or she has not. One US report estimated that false-positive readings might occur frequently with blood samples drawn from populations with a very low prevalence of HIV [14]. The frequency of such false-positive results is, however, heavily influenced by the skill and experience of the medical staff performing the analysis [15].

Testing in the tropics

But by far the greatest problem with false-positive results occurs in the tropics, where hot climates make unintentional bacterial contamination of blood samples more likely. Such samples are prone to give false results since they become "sticky", as does stored blood which has been repeatedly frozen and thawed.

Moreover, in rural tropical areas where people commonly suffer from multiple infections, such as malaria, schistosomiasis, tuberculosis or various worm infestations, problems of interpretation can make the accurate reading of HIV antibody tests very difficult. Because the immune systems of such multiply-infected people are in a chronically activated state, HIV antibody tests can be confounded by excessive antibody "noise".

In the mid-1980s testing for antibodies to HIV, which was carried out on African blood samples, generated a high percentage of false-positive results, leading to claims in some quarters that such tests were of little value in the African context.

The problem of ensuring accurate reading when testing "sticky" or "noisy" blood samples has been approached in different ways. A US approach is to subject samples which appear seropositive on the first test to a second, confirmatory test, usually one known as the Western Blot. Only samples which are shown to contain anti-HIV antibodies by both tests are considered to be truly positive.

The second approach is put forward mainly by British researchers. They agree that the US method of using two tests is better than one used alone, but think that the two US tests are too similar to rule out false-positive results on tricky blood samples, particularly in the tropics. The British approach employs not only two tests, but two very different types of test, so that any weakness in the first will be compensated by the second [16].

Testing blood for antibodies to the AIDS virus is a complicated business and, like any form of diagnostic test, there exists a margin of error in the results produced. Nevertheless, during the three years in which HIV antibody detection kits have been in use, improvements in their sensitivity and specificity have been made and this is as true of Africa as anywhere.

Antibody testing is expensive. A single test can cost between US$1 and US$5, with confirmatory tests running from US$30 to US$75 per patient. Laboratory and salary costs may add to the total. In the United States the testing of 3.2 million military recruits over two years has cost more than US$43 million [17]. Equipping just three laboratories to carry

HIV-antibody tests: some current developments

HIV-Chek (USA)
Advantages: Small, apparently accurate kit; test works rapidly. A drop of diluted blood produces a simple colour change. Laboratory unnecessary.
Disadvantages: Over US$4 per test: still too expensive for large-scale use in developing countries.

Haemagglutination test (Brazil)
Advantages: Produces result in 15 minutes with no special instrumentation. Said to have same sensitivity and specificity as the ELISA. At US$0.20 a test it could potentially find a large market.

Monoclonal antibody test (Canada)
Advantages: Simple, claimed to be accurate, can be used anywhere. Read by colour change; result in 10 minutes.
Disadvantages: At US$17 per test, far too expensive for use in developing countries.

Latex agglutination test (USA)
Advantages: Simple, no instrumentation required. Takes five minutes for result. African field trials have shown this test to be more accurate than a single ELISA test. No cost yet available.

Karpas cell test (Japan)
Advantages: New type of screening and confirmatory test taking two hours. Result read from a colour change. Suitable for use in developing countries and cheaper than current ELISA tests.

out blood screening over a three year period in Zaire will cost nearly US$2 million [18].

The trend in HIV antibody tests is toward simple, cheap, reliable kits whose results can be "read" on the spot, without much waiting and without the need for laboratory back-up. This box describes few of the most promising new tests.

HIV worsens other epidemics

If someone is infected in childhood with tuberculosis (TB), his or her immune system usually conquers the infection with no visible ill-effects, but may not completely eliminate the TB bacteria. The TB bacteria often remain dormant in the body, with the individual showing no signs of the disease, but nevertheless becoming a lifelong carrier. A TB carrier may remain well for life, or may develop active TB when his or her immune balance is upset — for example if infected by other organisms or if weakened through malnutrition.

TB is common in most Third World cities, and far more people are carriers than develop the lung disease which can end in coughing blood. Some 30-56% of adults in many developing countries probably have dormant TB infections [19].

When HIV infects a TB carrier, the resulting immune weakening can allow the TB bacteria to mount an active attack. If this attack is successful, the carrier then develops the lung or other tissue damage which can eventually be fatal.

But the chain of events does not end here. The tubercular patient has now become contagious, capable of passing on TB to his or her contacts — especially in damp, poorly-ventilated conditions.

So an epidemic of TB may be loosed in an apparently healthy community by a HIV-carrier showing no AIDS symptoms. The patient's doctor might see nothing but typical tuberculosis, and not think of testing for HIV — even if the test were available locally. WHO officials believe that AIDS may be the cause of the resurgence of TB presently occurring around the world.

In the United States the number of reported new TB cases rose by 2.6% in 1986, the first substantial increase in the lung disease among US citizens since the TB reporting system began in 1953 [20]. The incidence of TB had been declining by 7% annually between 1981 and 1984, years when the AIDS epidemic was in its early stages. In New York City, with nearly half the nation's reported AIDS cases, the incidence of TB increased by 35% in 1984-6.

Studies show close links between HIV and TB. Of 58 male tuberculosis patients in New York City, 31 were infected by HIV [21]. Forty per cent of TB patients tested in a study in Kinshasa, Zaire, were found to be HIV-carriers. In the same period, roughly 6-8% of healthy adults were HIV-positive [22]. And where TB infection is widespread, symptoms of tuberculosis are becoming more common among people in the 20-40 age group, the group most at risk from infection by HIV [23].

The experience of TB suggests that AIDS reflects and magnifies the infections that are prevalent in a particular locality [24]. Because diseases such as malaria and leprosy provoke strong immune reactions, WHO personnel with experience in tropical disease control speculate that other diseases could provoke a rapid downward spiral in the health of a person already infected with HIV [25]. They might trigger an active phase of HIV replication leading to the destruction of vital immune T-cells, leaving the person even more vulnerable to the ravages of malaria or leprosy.

Doctors report that HIV seems to exacerbate the damage done by the malarial parasite in the body. Malaria can cause brain damage in people whom the parasite has infected for the first time. Such damage is rare among adult Africans, but it now seems that people infected by HIV are more likely to suffer brain damage during recurrent bouts of malaria. Children especially may now be at risk from this more destructive form of an already damaging and common disease [26]. No one knows how HIV might interact with other diseases —

schistosomiasis (bilharzia), sleeping sickness, leishmaniasis — which are common in developing countries. By causing epidemics of infectious diseases besides AIDS, and by worsening the effects of other common infections, HIV poses a multiple challenge to health systems — and one which is likely to continue for many decades.

The role of genes: no firm evidence

Genetically-linked diseases do exist. Sickle cell anaemia, for example, which affects people in tropical Africa and less frequently in the Middle East and India, is caused by an inherited gene most commonly found among people of African racial groups. So the possibility that genes could also play a role in determining susceptibility to HIV or AIDS must be allowed. To a certain extent our individual genetic make-up, whatever racial group we happen to come from, always influences susceptibility to disease. But the question of whether certain racial groups might be more or less susceptible to AIDS is a highly controversial one.

Two groups of researchers, one in Britain and the other in Trinidad, have published data which suggested the possibility of a genetic factor in AIDS. Both sets of data have been criticised by other researchers, and neither has received much support in the scientific community. The British group recently found that its results had been mistaken, because of a previously undetectable malfunction in borrowed laboratory equipment which was used to perform their experiment. On discovering the malfunction the group quickly and formally withdrew its results, solving the mystery of why several other research teams were not able to duplicate them.

If, at some future time, susceptibility to AIDS does turn out to be influenced by genetic make-up, it is highly unlikely that there will be a genetic "switch" which works in an on-off fashion, making some individuals or ethnic groups vulnerable to AIDS and others immune. The role of genes is likely to be much more complex, with various genes interacting to modify the individual's vulnerability to infection by the AIDS virus, and the likelihood and speed of developing fatal AIDS, or interacting to vary the range of symptoms shown. Medical scientists have hardly begun to disentangle the multiple factors which may be involved.

Twin dangers: denial and delay

Almost every community in the world, when first confronted with the presence of the AIDS virus, has reacted by denying that the problem is real. Typically the cause or source of the disease is seen to lie somewhere

Overcoming denial

"One of the trickiest things about denial", says Richard Rector, a 31-year-old person with AIDS (PWA) who travels widely in both North and South as an AIDS educationalist, "is that at the time you usually don't realise that you're doing it". Rector relates how, in September 1986, he was one of 12 members of the board of directors of the US National Association of People With AIDS. By the end of October that year, there were only three others left. Eight members had died of AIDS in the interval.

"Throughout that two-month period I was in charge of the meetings and I would call them to order, proceeding through the agenda just as if nothing had happened. I wouldn't speak about or refer to the missing members. Then one day one of the remaining few blew up at me. 'You should stop this', he said. 'You are harming all of us by this behaviour.' They wanted to acknowledge those who had died and grieve for them, while I was steadfastly denying that anything unusual was happening.

"This may be hard to believe, but it's true, and it shows how deeply rooted is our tendency to deny things we feel we can't cope with. Because of this experience I can understand why so many countries have said

'We don't have AIDS, it's a Western disease', or 'We have AIDS, but it came from Africa', or whatever. Denial is a normal response and we must struggle both to recognise it is happening and to overcome it.

"What strikes me is that, until people are personally touched by AIDS, either by getting sick themselves or seeing friends or family members become seropositive, they just don't give a damn. They are content to fall back on all the old rationalisations that their own group or community is 'safe', and that someone else is at risk and at fault and deserving of, at best benign neglect and at worst punishment or forced isolation.

"PWAs have a special role to play in overcoming these attitudes. For one thing, they have crossed a certain fear threshold. They already have the disease which scares everyone half to death. They've had to learn to live with that fear and many of them have transcended it. Even though I'm a PWA myself, over and over again I've been impressed by how open and unafraid so many PWAs are. You can't help but be impressed. We can help people to learn to overcome the fear which blinds them to the realities of AIDS" **[29]**.

else. Thus, when AIDS cases first began to mount in the United States, an assumption was made that the infection must have arrived there from Haiti. Later on, popular opinion in the United States and in Europe had it that Africa was the source of AIDS, while in Africa, Europeans are often perceived as bringing in the infection. Among black and Latino people in the United States, AIDS has for some time been regarded as a white disease. In Japan, the Philippines and other parts of Asia, AIDS is often seen as a foreign disease, while many in Islamic countries believe that adherence to Koranic morality is sufficient protection from it.

Even among homosexual men in the United States, where AIDS struck early, hard, and in a blaze of publicity, denial reigned too long, according to those familiar with this community [27]. They argue that the fierce toll exacted by HIV on homosexual groups was in large measure a result of the unwillingness of homosexual men and others to face up to the truth of what was happening. And in the United Kingdom, where the virus arrived two or three years later than in the United States, precious lead time was lost to inaction while a minority of doctors vainly urged that a US-style epidemic could only be averted if denial was cast aside. It is important to recognise that denial is a typical human reaction to the threat of AIDS, because denial so often delays preventive action. Especially prior to the World Health Assembly in Geneva in May 1987, many governments delayed or prevented reports of AIDS cases from reaching WHO.

Newspapers in some African countries now openly acknowledge that for some time AIDS was something to keep quiet about. "A few years ago", said the *Times of Zambia* in August 1987, "there was an unwritten rule not to discuss the presence of AIDS in Zambia so as not to discourage tourists from coming here". According to the Nigerian magazine *Newswatch* in March 1987: "In the six years since the AIDS scourge spread across the world, Nigeria has tried its best to wish it away". Not until 1987 did US President Ronald Reagan make a public statement on his country's epidemic [28]. Blame and denial, which have seriously undermined action against AIDS, are discussed more fully in Chapter Six, and in the Panos book *Blaming Others: prejudice, race and worldwide AIDS* (London and Washington DC, 1988).

CHAPTER TWO

ANY TREATMENT?
ANY CURE?

Diseases caused by viruses can be relatively harmless (like the common cold), or lethal (like smallpox). Viruses may produce symptoms a short time after infection (as is the case with influenza), or may take decades to produce a fatal disease (like leukaemia).

At the end of the Second World War, only a handful of human viruses were known. Hundreds more have been discovered since, partly as a result of advanced techniques for culturing them in the laboratory. Viruses are parasites which infect almost every form of life, from single-celled bacteria up to humans. They can only live and grow inside the cells of another "host" organism, such as the human body.

In evolutionary terms, host and virus populations engage in skirmishes which most often result in the elimination of the viral infection by the host's immune system. Influenza, measles and polio are examples of viral disease which, more often than not, our bodies combat successfully, rendering us immune to subsequent infection by the same virus. These diseases have short incubation periods of days or weeks between infection and the appearance of symptoms, and the symptoms themselves are generally short-lived. In order to maintain its existence within the host community, the virus must pass from infected to uninfected individuals within this short period, or risk being eliminated as an increasing number of hosts develop protective immunity. The virus in this case requires a very large host population in order to survive: in the case of measles in excess of 100,000 individuals.

In certain other types of illness, however, the virus employs a different survival strategy. After infecting the host and triggering an initial acute bout of symptoms, viruses such as those of the herpes family stop producing any obvious sickness and become latent, living unnoticed in the host's cells for months or years until conditions are right for the triggering of another acute outburst of symptoms. Called latent viruses, they can survive in small host populations by making their hosts periodically infective during the acute phases of the illness.

A third viral survival strategy features aspects of the above two approaches. Combining infectivity which lasts for much of the duration of the illness (as with measles), with persistence in the host's body long after the first symptoms appear (as with herpes), viruses like those causing Hepatitis B and AIDS seem to cause lifelong infections, *'if you are infected with the AIDS virus, you will almost certainly go on to get AIDS'* during which time the host is thought to be capable of transmitting the virus to others. These viruses are called "slow viruses" or lentiviruses. They are rare and belong to a larger group of viruses known as the *retroviruses*. Human retroviruses are a relatively new discovery.

Persistent viral infections can be sustained over long periods of time in small host communities. They can, in theory at least, be spread to a new and uninfected host population by a single carrier. When the disease they cause breaks out, with deceptive suddenness, months or years later, it may well be impossible to trace how or when the infection was first introduced. This persistence explains why the exact event which marks the beginning of an AIDS epidemic in a given community can so rarely be identified, but it does not explain where the AIDS virus came from in the first place. What is known about the origins of the AIDS virus is discussed in Chapter Three.

Does HIV always kill?

By 1988 doctors had been aware of AIDS for barely seven years. Most of the careful statistical research on survival with AIDS goes back barely five years. This is not long enough to study an infection which can remain "silent" for 5-10 years or more.

Over the past two years or so a mass of seemingly contradictory data on the survival chances of HIV-positive individuals has appeared. Much of the apparent lack of consistency may be due to the fact that the statistical studies which have been done use different methodologies and different sizes of sample groups, and vary in the way they sort the various symptoms of HIV infection into diagnostic categories such as PGL, AIDS-related complex and AIDS.

While US health authorities still officially estimate that only 20-30% of seropositives will develop AIDS within five years, other studies have yielded gloomier results. Researchers at San Francisco General Hospital have followed a group of 288 homosexual men, most of whom are believed to have been infected by HIV in 1981-2. Based on three years of study, the researchers predict that six years from the date of infection 50% of the study group will have developed AIDS and an additional 25% will experience AIDS-related symptoms [1]. Interpreting the results, the lead researcher told reporters: "What we saw was that the number of those showing no effects from HIV infection is very small. This means that if you are infected with the AIDS virus, you will almost certainly go on to get AIDS" [2].

Another San Francisco study of 63 homosexual men whose dates of infection could be pinpointed showed that 30% developed AIDS within seven years [3]. And scientists at Frankfurt University in West Germany found that of a group of 543 people (most of them the sexual partners of people with AIDS) studied since 1982, only 9.8% of the HIV-carriers remained healthy after three years. Using computer modelling these researchers predicted that 50% of HIV carriers will develop AIDS within five years, and 75% within seven years [4].

Evidence from the US Walter Reed Army Medical Center indicates that 80-90% of all HIV-infected individuals experience some level of deterioration in their immune system over a few years, suggesting that the vast majority of them "will be adversely affected by the virus over time" [5].

The unanswered question is: will the percentage of infected individuals who become ill keep rising until it approaches 100%, or will it start to level off at some future point in time? "The final toll is unknown", says Dr Anthony Fauci, director of the US National Institute of Allergy and Infectious Diseases [6]. Dr Richard Tedder, one of Britain's leading virologists, is pessimistic about the prospects, believing that ultimately a very high percentage of the people infected with HIV may die of AIDS. "But with a virus of this type and long latency period," he adds, "a proportion of seropositive individuals may not manifest symptoms for a decade or decades. Slow virus infections are such that a person's natural lifespan may be reached before the onset of disease. Only time will allow us to determine if this is the case with HIV" [7].

In its latest report the US National Academy of Sciences states that, over time, "a larger and larger proportion of seropositive persons has been seen to develop AIDS. The data are now available to suggest that the great majority of HIV-infected persons will eventually progress to AIDS in the absence of effective therapy to slow or halt the progression of the infection" [8].

Furthermore, the US report recommends that HIV infection should itself be considered a disease. The prevalence of HIV infection is just as important as the incidence of AIDS, the report says, and it goes on to urge that policymakers include both HIV infection and AIDS in their assessment of the scale and scope of the epidemic. From a public health point of view, the report's authors argue, "the important event is infection rather than full-blown disease because even asymptomatic infected individuals are capable of infecting others".

Other prominent researchers have speculated that a range of diverse factors may affect the progression of HIV infection to AIDS. Some suggest that the greater the original infecting dose of HIV, the worse are the individual's chances of remaining healthy [9]. Some believe that the particular strain of virus contracted by an individual has an influence [10]. Laboratory evidence lends support to the belief that some strains of the AIDS virus are more virulent than others, perhaps causing the people infected by them to become ill and die more quickly. French researchers have isolated a Zairean strain of the AIDS virus, which they call HIV-NDK, which, they say, kills human cells faster than strains of HIV from the United States or Europe [11].

Some AIDS physicians and their patients work on the assumption that the "lifestyle" of the infected person — subsequent exposure to other infections, diet, exercise and mental attitude, and use of drugs, alcohol, or other toxic substances — play an important role in determining whether a latent HIV infection progresses to AIDS [12].

A study of 5,833 AIDS patients in New York City suggests that the health environment of the seropositive person could well play a role in determining the ultimate outcome of HIV infection even after AIDS has developed. Of these patients, male and female and drawn from different racial, social, age and diagnostic groups, 15% survived for five years. The long survivors were more likely to be younger, male and white, and to have had Kaposi's sarcoma rather than pneumocystis

Surviving with AIDS

In May 1983 Louis Nassaney of San Diego, California, 33 years old, was diagnosed with Kaposi's sarcoma and given six months to live. Five years later he told the London *Sunday Times*: "I feel as healthy now as I was before Aids — in fact, more healthy" [14].

Nassaney is only one of a number of individuals in the United States, Britain and other countries who are surviving much longer than the average 18 months after diagnosis of AIDS. Several factors appear linked to better survival times. The longest-lived group in one New York study were homosexual men in their thirties who had Kaposi's sarcoma and no other opportunistic infection. Black women who acquired AIDS through intravenous drug use had the shortest survival time [15].

It seems that those who live longest do so for a variety of reasons. They have access to better health care, which means not only better treatment but earlier diagnosis. They have a positive self-image, a will to survive and the encouragement and support of family and friends. They adjust their diets to eliminate alcohol, caffeine and artificial foods, while eating more fresh fruit and other healthy foods.

Many long-term survivors have either rejected conventional medicine or complemented it with "alternative" treatments such as homeopathy or acupuncture. The philosophy underlying such treatments is to approach not only the symptoms of AIDS but the patient's general well-being, including their personal relationships, emotions and attitude to life.

People who survive for a long time with AIDS appear to have been successful in building their own individual support network of friends, alternative healers, PWA groups, psychological and spiritual advisors and others, drawing on what they feel is useful in their own particular case and rejecting the rest.

So far there is little research and thus little evidence that diet and "alternative" treatments do enable people with AIDS to live longer. A key factor could be psychological: people survive if they believe they are going to do so, and planning their own treatment routine promotes this belief.

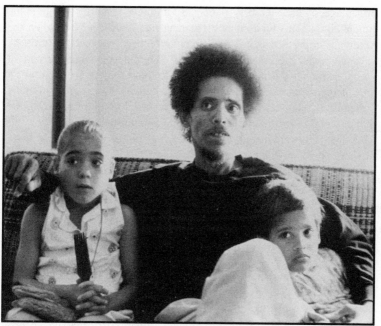

Figure 2.1
Father, son and
daughter in a New
York clinic, where
all three are being
treated for HIV
infection; the father
and son have since
died. So far,
treatment is very
expensive, and at
best slows down the
development of
AIDS. Poorer access
to health care means
that after diagnosis
with AIDS a black
or Latino man in the
United States lives
for only one fifth the
time of a white male
adult.

Curt Kaufman

pneumonia. Increasing age, female sex, black or Latino ethnicity, and having had pneumocystis pneumonia (common among intravenous drug users) were all factors which shortened survival [13].

In the United States the average lifespan of a white person after diagnosis with AIDS is about two years. From diagnosis the average black or Latino person with AIDS survives only 28 weeks [16]. Comparatively few doctors work in minority communities; fewer of their patients have health insurance, and they are both socially and financially less likely to seek early treatment. Minority patients are likely to be less healthy than their white counterparts before they contract the virus, a fact relating to their lower socio-economic status. By the time they present themselves for treatment their symptoms are already far advanced.

If these social, economic and behavioural factors can affect the survival time after AIDS diagnosis, they may also influence whether and how quickly HIV infection progresses to AIDS.

Treatments for AIDS

Seven years after its first diagnosis in the United States, there is still no cure for AIDS. But treatment *is* improving, and consists mainly of fighting the symptoms of the "opportunistic" infections which take advantage of the victim's damaged immune system: pneumonia, fungal infection, tuberculosis, cancer and diarrhoea. But when the treatment stops, the same or a different infection eventually returns. A substance which eliminated the virus without poisoning the patient would be the ideal drug for treating AIDS, but even this would not be a cure if the virus had already destroyed part of the person's immune system. In this case curing the patient would require repairing the damage and restoring immune functioning to normal.

As yet there are no antiviral drugs which permanently rid the body of HIV. There are two reasons:

- HIV "hides" in the body cells it infects. To kill it, a drug will also probably kill these cells, damaging the patient's immune system even more.

- The virus can infect brain cells, where most antiviral drugs cannot follow, because they are "filtered out" by the blood-brain barrier. It is extremely difficult to design a drug that will enter the brain and kill the HIV without damaging the brain itself.

Instead of focusing on antiviral agents, much research is now being directed towards drugs which prevent the virus from reproducing and colonising more immune system cells. AIDS patients would have to take these drugs for life; unfortunately many of the drugs tested so far have toxic side effects, even in the short term.

The development of a new chemical or biological substance to be used as a drug treatment for specific diseases is, in most countries, a lengthy, expensive and highly regulated process. Pharmaceutical companies normally spend many years and invest tens or hundreds of millions of dollars to bring a new drug through the research, testing, licensing and finally marketing stages of development. In the United States the process, regulated by the Food and Drug Administration, can take a decade or more. It is designed to ensure that all licensed drugs are of proven use, have no unexpected side effects and are not poisonous.

Because new drugs take so long to develop, most of the drugs currently thought to have potential as AIDS treatments are a decade or more old, and were originally developed to combat other diseases. A good deal of AIDS research consists of screening old drugs for use against the new threat. Having been through the licensing process of testing on animals, small groups of humans and then large groups of patients, these drugs must nevertheless demonstrate their effectiveness on groups of AIDS patients before they can be routinely prescribed by doctors. AIDS patients in the United States, frustrated by the length of time it has taken to license AIDS drugs, have lobbied to speed up the process. One result has been that the state of California has established its own system to test and possibly approve new AIDS drugs [17].

Some critics of the present system of drug research argue that much more could and should be done to screen existing drugs and therapies for their usefulness in treating AIDS. But, they say, pharmaceutical companies are more interested in developing new drugs for which they can obtain the exclusive legal patents which ensure maximum profitability. Existing drugs which show potential are not being researched, maintain these critics, and worse, "many medical researchers are demonstrably aligned through financial support with the drug companies whose efforts they are supposed to police" [18].

At present the leader in the field of AIDS drugs is *zidovudine*, commonly known as AZT, and sold under the trade name Retrovir. (Zidovudine was formerly known as azidothymidine or AZT, and since this is the most widely recognised name for this drug, it is the one which is used throughout this dossier.) AZT crosses the blood-brain barrier, can be taken orally, and has been approved for use against AIDS in most industrialised countries. In certain classes of AIDS patients it seems to improve immunologic functioning and may partially reverse nervous system damage [19].

But AZT is toxic to bone marrow even at low doses, causing severe anaemia, with over a quarter of patients requiring blood transfusions [20]. British researchers have found that, despite its benefits, it causes side effects ranging from nausea, loss of appetite and insomnia to severe anaemia, lung complications, and toxic interactions with other drugs — reactions severe enough to lead to death. They also found that when they reduced AZT doses in order to prevent toxic reactions, the AIDS virus was reactivated, causing a patient to die [21].

Despite the side effects, AZT is credited with prolonging the lives of a sufficient number of AIDS patients that it is now being tried on people infected with HIV before they show symptoms of AIDS, in the hope that it may prevent the disease from developing [22]. AZT has been around since the 1960s, when it was developed as a drug to combat cancer. It is made from thymidine, a substance extracted from the sperm of herring and salmon. Burroughs-Wellcome, the transnational company which manufactures AZT under the brand name Retrovir, has reportedly cornered the market on thymidine by acquiring rights to all of the limited amount of the substance which can currently be made [23] — thus securing its position as a monopoly producer of the only AIDS drug so far licensed.

This monopoly position is one reason, people with AIDS have argued, that Retrovir costs in the region of US$10,000 per year per patient. The drug is so expensive that some US doctors say that AIDS

'many AIDS patients have been driven into destitution' patients in the United States and Europe are treating themselves with drugs obtained illegally, either from "pirate" laboratories or by smuggling them in from other countries [24]. A number of groups of people with AIDS in the United States believe that the price of AZT is five to ten times greater than the actual cost of manufacturing the drug. They allege that Burroughs-Wellcome is attempting to make as much money as it can out of AZT before another, less toxic, drug arrives on the scene and reduces its market. Burroughs-Wellcome and other manufacturers who have useful drugs have "raised the prices to the maximum the market of terrified people will stand", say AIDS activists, and many AIDS patients "have been driven into destitution [25]".

A drug which is considered to be as promising as AZT is Ampligen, a decoy virus which stimulates the immune system resulting in increased activity against HIV. Ampligen crosses the blood-brain barrier, and has helped patients with symptoms both of AIDS and ARC [26]. But like AZT, if licensed it will be extremely expensive. Drugs (as yet) unapproved for AIDS treatment, but in current use, include:

- Imuthiol, a drug developed and available, at a cost, from the Institut Merieux Lyons, in France;
- DDC (dideoxycitidine), like AZT a failed cancer drug, which is being studied in the United States, but is not yet approved;
- Ribavirin, a viral inhibitor available in Mexico, which showed little promise in limited human trials, but on which further testing is to take place;
- AL721, a drug developed in Israel, made from egg yolk and which, some people with AIDS argue, should be classed as a food supplement and not required to go through the drug licensing procedure;
- Dextran sulphate, an anti-viral agent which may have benefit when combined with AZT and is currently in early trials.

With the exception of AL721, all these drugs, and others which have been named as possible AIDS treatments, have one thing in common: if successfully brought to market they are likely to be very expensive, prohibitively so in the Third World. Can the HIV-damaged immune system be repaired, or its cells replaced, restoring the AIDS patient's resistance to infections? Use of biological substances such as the repair treatments interferon and interleukin-2, and immune replacements including lymphocyte transfusions, bone marrow transplants and thymic implants, have been tried on a few patients with some success.

Recently a novel treatment has been proposed: a natural protein which would "soak up" the AIDS virus in infected people. The substance is a human protein, CD4, which sits on the surface of immune system cells, and which the AIDS virus is attracted to as it seeks to infect these cells. US researchers think that if CD4 is administered to people already infected, the protein might serve as a decoy, absorbing the virus and halting its spread to new cells. It might also be possible to attach virus-killing drugs to the protein in order to deliver them directly to the AIDS virus [27].

In the final resort though, treatments that do not eliminate the HIV virus from the body are only temporary victories. Ideally, a combination of anti-viral and immune repair/replacement treatments may within a

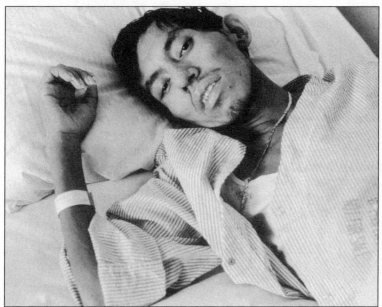

Alon Reininger/ Contact/ Colourific

Figure 2.2
So far, drug treatments for AIDS are only partly effective—and far too expensive for widespread Third World use. This Latino man, a former seaman in the US Navy in a veterans hospital, is more fortunate than many illegal immigrants to the United States. Even if they have been US residents for some years, US law requires that those who are HIV-positive when they apply for citizenship be sent back to their country of origin, where their chances of treatment are remote and they may spread HIV infection further.

few years offer better results. But there is no doubt that such sophisticated treatments will be too expensive for most of the world's HIV-carriers, who live in developing countries.

Drug research is beginning to take an even higher priority as hopes for an early AIDS vaccine fade. Many researchers are optimistic that combinations of drugs and other therapies will, in the not too distant future, allow people with HIV and AIDS to live a nearly normal life. But treatments for HIV and AIDS, like those for chronic diseases such as diabetes, will have to be prolonged for the lifetime of the patient *'in 1988 research suffered major setbacks'* — over which time cumulative side-effects will have to be minimised if the treatments are to be useful.

The body defends itself against viruses by using its lymphocytes to produce virus-killing cells and antibodies. This natural defence does not work against HIV.

One way of "artificially" protecting the body against viruses is to use a vaccine: either a dose of killed virus, or a dose of a mild strain of the live virus. Neither dose is sufficient to cause illness, but both will stimulate the lymphocytes to produce appropriate antibodies themselves.

AIDS vaccine: early hopes diminish

Can this be done with HIV to immunise uninfected people against AIDS? When the second edition of this dossier was published in March 1987, a climate of cautious optimism reigned among scientists engaged in AIDS vaccine research. While a few virologists were more pessimistic, the consensus was that an effective vaccine would be available within a decade or so. In mid-1987 encouragement was supplied by the results of a vaccine experiment conducted in Zaire. French doctor Daniel Zagury and Zairean volunteers inoculated themselves with a vaccine preparation which they found stimulated some of their immune systems to produce antibodies against HIV [28].

What was lacking after this and other experiments was evidence that the antibodies produced would offer protection against HIV infection. To find out if this were the case, it would be necessary to expose the subjects in whom antibody production had been stimulated to the AIDS virus — a critical and potentially dangerous step which researchers are still not ready to take.

Intermediate between this hazardous step and research such as that of the Zairean group is experimentation on animals which can be infected with AIDS viruses and which develop an antibody response against them. But early in 1988 animal research suffered major setbacks. Chimpanzees given doses of a type of antibody that neutralises HIV in laboratory dishes were not protected against infection when they were subsequently inoculated with AIDS viruses. In another trial monkeys were vaccinated with inactivated preparations of a monkey virus which causes an illness similar to AIDS. The monkeys had an excellent antibody response, but were completely unprotected against later AIDS infection [29]. One of the leading US vaccine researchers commented that the animal failures were "real setbacks and they raise serious concerns about the viability of the vaccine programme" [30].

In mid-1988 it is still impossible to say whether the setbacks are temporary, or whether they signal that the road to an effective vaccine will be much longer than anyone has anticipated.

Meanwhile vaccine research carries on, with testing of various potentially immunising preparations involving human subjects getting the go-ahead in both the United States and Britain.

Developing a vaccine against AIDS is complicated by the variability of the AIDS virus: a vaccine that works against one strain of HIV may not give protection against others. There are a number of possible approaches that take this and other problems into account. The first approach is the possibility that specific protein sub-parts of the AIDS virus might be made into a vaccine which would trigger both antibody and killer-cell response. A number of variants on this approach are being tried:

- An AIDS vaccine might be made from the protein "skin" or envelope of the HIV virus. Researchers have discovered that a portion of the envelope — the signature protein — may remain unchanged from strain to strain. If this portion of the envelope could be separated, its genes could then be spliced into the harmless vaccinia virus used in the smallpox vaccine, to create an HIV vaccine. This was the approach adopted by Dr Zagury and colleagues in Zaire.

- A synthetic envelope protein of the AIDS virus might be genetically engineered in the laboratory, and then made into an injectable preparation. A US biotechnology company, which has succeeded in producing such a synthetic protein, has received permission to try it on humans, and is currently recruiting volunteers on which to test its effectiveness in triggering immune response [31].

- A US-British group is working on a vaccine made from a protein found just below the surface of the virus, because it is not as susceptible to variation between strains as the surface proteins. The group has genetically engineered the protein and will soon test the vaccine on human volunteers [32].

A second approach might be to produce a vaccine which would target the core of HIV, since the core genes appear to vary less than those for the envelope. This is being tried, with results from trials on rabbits, dogs and monkeys showing that an immune response was produced.

A third approach involves the use of substances which might prevent the AIDS virus from infecting body cells by blocking their point of entry [33].

A fourth approach would be to use the whole AIDS virus, rather than a natural or genetically engineered sub-unit of it, as a basis for a vaccine. Of course, the AIDS virus would first have to be killed or inactivated to deprive it of its infective and cell-destroying capabilities. A proponent of this approach is Dr Jonas Salk, the scientist who developed the first *'to deny a vaccine might be genocide'*

vaccine against polio in the 1950s.   The AIDS virus is killed by irradiating it, and its injection into laboratory monkeys has stimulated a good antibody response.

Its potential benefit is that by using the whole AIDS virus in a vaccine, the immune system would be stimulated to produce a range of antibodies against different viral proteins, a response which might provide greater protection than if antibodies were produced to a single selected viral protein. But some researchers fear that this idea will backfire by overstimulating the immune system and causing it to wear down, making it even more susceptible to AIDS than would otherwise be the case [34].

If the first phase of human vaccine trials currently under way produce a promising candidate vaccine, the next stage in the research would pose formidable practical and ethical problems. Who would be the first to be tested? How would the effectiveness of the vaccine be ascertained in a period of time shorter than the full HIV incubation period of five to ten years or more? The sexual behaviour of those vaccinated would have to be closely monitored for years. There might be severe side effects. To develop a set of internationally applicable guidelines for the testing of AIDS vaccines is a task for WHO, which has played a similar role with respect to other infectious diseases. (For a discussion of the need for such guidelines see Chapter Eight.)

After human trials, the delivery of the vaccine would be highly complex. Drug companies might not be anxious to market the new product: there would be immense potential for expensive lawsuits [35]. What would the new vaccine cost? Could it be distributed on a mass scale, or would only selective high-risk groups be chosen for inoculation? Who would do the choosing? Would distribution in Third World countries be more difficult?

In Haiti and several African countries nearly everyone might have to be vaccinated; the expense would be enormous. But to deny such a vaccine might be considered genocide. The vaccine against Hepatitis B, which has become available over the past year, provides an example of just how costly such bio-engineered products can be.

This hepatitis vaccine is not "manufactured" like a drug, but "grown", like a microbial culture. Laboratory growing of the microorganisms used in a vaccine takes a lot of time, expensive equipment and materials, and immense skill. At present it costs about US$180 per person to immunise against Hepatitis B. An AIDS vaccine is likely to be similarly costly, at least in the first years of development, which would make its mass use in poor countries problematic.

And it must be stressed that a vaccine could only stop new people being infected with the HIV virus. It would have no effect on the tens of millions who by then will probably be HIV-positive.

CHAPTER THREE

THE AIDS PANDEMIC

The virus which causes AIDS is one of the nastiest microbes ever to have hit humankind.

The disease it causes seems to be virtually always fatal; the virus may give no sign of its presence for years; there is so far no vaccine and no cure; and it is mainly spread from person to person by sexual contact.

But there is one "good" thing to say about the AIDS virus: relatively speaking, it is not very infectious. Unlike influenza or tuberculosis, it is not spread by coughs and sneezes; unlike malaria or plague, it is not carried by insects; unlike cholera, it is not carried in contaminated food or water; unlike smallpox, you cannot catch it by casual skin contact.

Transmission methods are discussed more fully in Chapter five. In general, the virus can be passed from one person to another:

- by penetrative sexual contact (vaginal, anal and possibly oral)
- by sharing unsterilised hypodermic needles, on the part of by intravenous drug users (ivdu) or careless medical personnel
- by a blood transfusion with contaminated blood
- by contaminated blood products
- by transplanted organs or donated semen
- by blood from an infected person entering another's cut or wound: as a result of tattooing, or as may occur in ritual tribal scarring or circumcision, or in traditional medicine or other circumstances where cutting or piercing implements are shared
- from mother to baby before, during and possibly after birth.

The growth of the pandemic

By the end of 1981, the year in which AIDS was first diagnosed, 180 cases had been reported by the US Centers for Disease Control (CDC); six months later CDC had reported 403 cases from 24 of the 50 US states. Around this time 200 AIDS cases had been noted in Europe, 42 of them in people of African origin who had travelled to Europe for treatment [1].

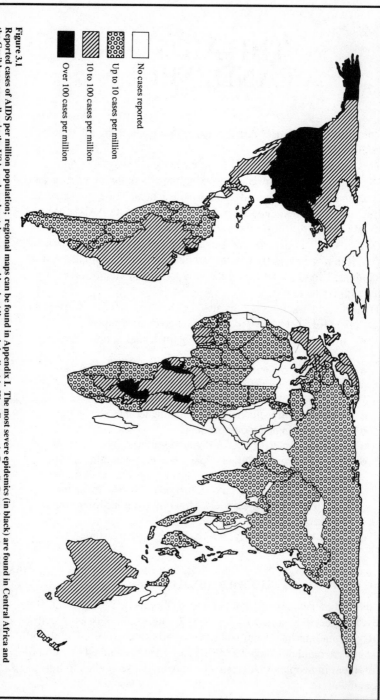

Figure 3.1
Reported cases of AIDS per million population; regional maps can be found in Appendix I. The most severe epidemics (in black) are found in Central Africa and the Caribbean as well as in the USA, and moderately severe epidemics (diagonal shading) in West Europe, in Brazil, Central America, Mexico and Canada, in parts of Africa, and in Australia and New Zealand. Like all the maps in this dossier, this one uses the Peters projection, which indicates the true relative area of each country. The actual number of AIDS cases may be larger than those officially reported, and some countries in which AIDS is present do not report at all and therefore appear blank on the map. Source: Panos, from WHO figures and other official reports up to June 1988.

No cases reported

Up to 10 cases per million

10 to 100 cases per million

Over 100 cases per million

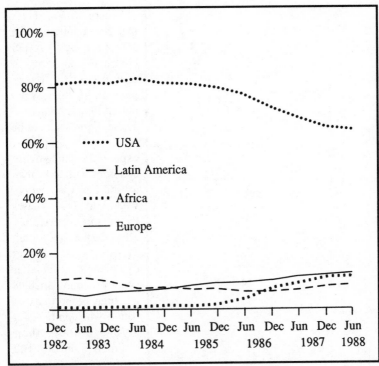

Figure 3.2
As more and more
AIDS cases are
reported from
outside the United
States, the US share
of the global
epidemic has fallen
steadily from just
over 80% in 1983/4
to about 65% in
mid-1988.
Source: Panos,
based on WHO
figures.

By the end of 1982 WHO had reports of 1,668 cases of AIDS in 17 countries in the Americas and Europe, with only three countries outside these regions (South Africa, Israel and Australia) reporting cases. One year later 29 countries reported a cumulative world total of 5,096 cases, three times the previous year's number. Although several African countries were already heavily affected by AIDS, only Rwanda had reported cases of the disease to WHO by the end of 1983.

During 1984 a third African country (the Central African Republic) and a second Asian country (Thailand) began reporting AIDS cases, which by the end of the year had more than doubled to a global total of 12,030. Another doubling occurred in 1985, bringing the cumulative world total to 24,591 cases reported by 33 American, 20 European, six African and nine Asian/Oceania countries. The cumulative global total nearly doubled again in 1986 (45,966 cases reported by 102 countries), reached 73,747 cases by the end of 1987 (reported from 129 countries). By the end of June 1988 the total had climbed to 100,410 cases in 138 of the 176 countries reporting to WHO.

Early in 1988 the United States had 65% of all the AIDS cases reported to the WHO. But a number of Third World countries are, in per capita terms, considerably worse off.

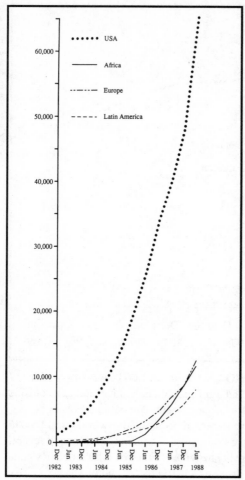

Figure 3.3
Although the bulk of
reported AIDS cases
reported to WHO
are from the United
States, cases
reported from
Africa, Europe and
Latin America are
also rising steeply.
Source: WHO.

Figure 3.4 shows the 20 countries most affected by AIDS epidemics, in terms of cumulative cases reported to the WHO per million population. These figures should be read with caution, especially those from countries with less than a million population, where a few cases can disproportionately affect the per capita total. Moreover, the number of cases in smaller countries may include a high proportion of people who contracted it abroad and then returned home. The figures may also be misleading in that in the United States and in some African countries, AIDS cases are heavily concentrated in major cities, and not spread throughout rural areas.

Nevertheless, it is clear that in per capita terms a number of Third World countries already have statistically more severe AIDS epidemics than does the United States. AIDS epidemics appear to be most serious in Africa, the Caribbean, Europe and North America — with 18 of the top 20 countries in Africa and the Caribbean.

Are AIDS cases reported accurately?

There are a variety of logistical, economic and political reasons for supposing that official figures, especially those from the Third World, significantly underestimate the real position. WHO estimates that, worldwide to the end of 1987, only about half of all AIDS cases had been reported to it.

Figure 3.4

COUNTRIES MOST AFFECTED BY AIDS
IN TERMS OF REPORTED CASES PER CAPITA

	Officially reported cases	National population	A I D S cases per million population
French Guiana	113	82,000	1,378
Bermuda	75	56,000	1,339
Bahamas	188	235,000	800
Congo	1,250	2,100,000	595
USA	65,780	243,800,000	270
Guadeloupe	74	300,000	247
Burundi	1,156	5,000,000	231
Haiti	1,374	6,200,000	222
Barbados	55	300,000	183
Trinidad	227	1,300,000	175
Uganda	2,369	15,900,000	149
Rwanda	901	6,800,000	133
Martinique	38	300,000	127
Qatar	32	300,000	107
Zambia	754	7,100,000	106
St Lucia	10	100,000	100
Central African Rep	254	2,700,000	94
Netherlands Antilles	18	200,000	90
Malawi	583	7,400,000	79
Dominican Rep	504	6,500,000	78

Source: Panos, based on national and WHO figures officially reported by June 1988, excluding countries reporting fewer than 10 cases.

A few countries do not report AIDS cases at all, although the number of non-reporting countries decreased dramatically during 1987 and early 1988. In developing countries, where medical surveillance systems are often weak, many, perhaps the majority, of AIDS cases are not reported to the national health authorities. In the United States, analyses suggest that about 90% of the AIDS cases meeting the official WHO criteria are actually reported [2]. In some areas of Europe

'150,000 will develop AIDS in 1988' as many as 50% of cases may go unreported [3]. Pan American Health Organization officials believe that in Latin America between 10% and 50% of AIDS cases are not reported [4]. Moreover, in many countries North and South some doctors will diagnose pneumonia, cancer or another opportunistic infection rather than AIDS, to avoid stigmatising either the patient or the patient's family.

According to WHO and other authorities, "reporting of AIDS cases in Africa has in general been delayed or incomplete", due to "limited access of large segments of the population to health care facilities where the diagnosis of AIDS can be established, the low efficiency of surveillance systems, the general lack of facilities for the diagnosis of AIDS, and the reluctance of some governments to acknowledge the existence of AIDS until 1987" [5]. AIDS statistics, particularly in Africa, where the false results of early blood test surveys have muddied the waters, remain an extremely sensitive issue politically, as do claims by Westerners that rates of underreporting on the continent are high.

A sense of proportion

No one knows how many people have died thus far of AIDS, though WHO estimates that by the end of 1987 150,000 cases of the disease had probably occurred worldwide [6]. A further 150,000 people will develop AIDS in 1988, and by 1991 WHO expects that one million people will have fallen ill [7]. In the United States the death toll reached 65,000 by June 1988. Research in New York City suggests that even in the United States, which has one of the strongest disease surveillance systems in the world, AIDS cases and deaths have been underestimated by 10% or more [8]. In Western Europe 4,640 AIDS deaths have been recorded, probably an underestimate. In Africa, WHO estimates that 10,000 people each year may be dying of AIDS [9].

Though they represent tremendous suffering, these figures are dwarfed by the numbers of people who die every day, especially in the Third World, from entirely preventable causes. If 75,000 people have died of AIDS since the pandemic began, a quarter of a million children die *each week* from the quiet carnage of undernourishment and preventable infection [10]. Worldwide, one in every three deaths is of a child under five years of age — a total of 14 million children each year. Statistics such as these have prompted some health professionals to caution against overreaction to the AIDS pandemic, and to warn that excessive attention to AIDS could suck resources away from existing and vital areas of health care.

Their argument is an important one, but it must be balanced against the fact that the AIDS pandemic is still in its infancy. The number of deaths so far may be relatively small compared to other causes of

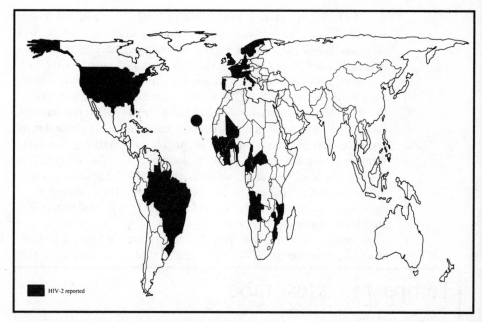

HIV-2 reported

mortality in the developing world, but the true death toll will only be known in the years to come, as those already silently infected by the AIDS virus fall ill. WHO's estimate is that between five and ten million people may already be infected [11], and that up to 100 million could contract the virus by the end of the century.

Two AIDS viruses

It is often confusing to talk of "the AIDS virus", because there are now two separate viruses which have been connected with AIDS: HIV-1 and HIV-2.

HIV-1 (formerly known as HTLV-3 or LAV) is associated with epidemics in central, east and southern Africa, in North and South America, Europe and the rest of the world. It leads to AIDS in half or more of the people it infects.

HIV-2 is often called the second AIDS virus and was originally named LAV-2 by its French discoverers. It has been isolated from both healthy and AIDS-affected people in several west African countries. It is not yet certain whether HIV-2 will cause an AIDS epidemic in West Africa of similar magnitude to that caused in central Africa and the rest of the world by HIV-1.

Doctors have not yet been able to establish whether AIDS patients infected by HIV-2 will suffer the same disease symptoms as those infected by HIV-1. Epidemiological evidence lends support to the belief

Figure 3.5
By June 1988, the "second" AIDS virus HIV-2 had been reported from Africa, Europe, North and South America. It appears to cause similar symptoms of AIDS as does HIV-1, and has the potential to grow into as serious a global epidemic.
Source: Panos

that the HIV-2 epidemic is quite recent, and only time will tell how it will develop. This relationship, and the origins of the monkey virus discussed below (see box: Tempest in a test tube), have for three years generated much heated debate among scientists and non-scientists alike.

HIV-2 was discovered in 1986, and reported to be present in three west African countries — Cape Verde, Guinea-Bissau and Senegal — by the French researchers who isolated it from AIDS patients [12]. Now fairly widespread in these countries and in the Ivory Coast [13], its presence has also been reported in Angola [14], Burkina Faso [15], Cameroon [16], the Central African Republic [17], the Gambia [18], Guinea [19], Mali [20] and Mozambique [21]. HIV-2 appears to cause AIDS symptoms very similar to those caused by HIV-1, though more time and experience with the second AIDS virus is needed to establish the clinical pattern of disease it provokes.

Scientists working on HIV-2 believe that it has the same epidemic potential as HIV-1. The reason that more cases of AIDS

Tempest in a test tube

Early in 1983 a primate research centre in California reported four outbreaks of an AIDS-like disease in captive monkeys [28]. Later the monkeys were found to be infected by a virus which, on inspection, showed similarities to the AIDS virus [29]. The original source of this monkey virus, called SIV (simian — for monkey — immunodeficiency virus), is at present unknown, a fact which raises many questions.

Why should captive monkeys carry a virus similar to the AIDS virus (HIV-1) which has infected millions of people around the world? Where did the captive monkeys contract their virus? Could they have been infected in their natural habitat, before their capture? Or is it more likely that they were infected by cage-mate monkeys of their own, or another species or even, perhaps, by humans? The incomplete state of research into some of these these questions has left room for a great deal of confusion.

When, in 1985-6, two US scientists endeavoured to trace the origins of SIV to monkeys living in the wild, they focused their

researches on West Africa. There they thought they had found not one but two new AIDS-like viruses, a discovery which generated enormous publicity. The two scientists, working with French and Senegalese colleagues, thought they had isolated a new virus from wild African green monkeys, and a second very similar virus from people living in Senegal. Their findings appeared to confirm a theory about the origins of the AIDS virus: that it had sprung into existence in Africa, passed from monkeys to humans there, and been carried from there to other parts of the world.

This theory about the origins of AIDS caused much anger and distress among many groups of Africans who felt, first, that the world was unjustly concluding that their continent had somehow started a worldwide epidemic; and second, that this conclusion was based on flimsy, even biased, evidence. From 1985 onwards bitter controversy over the "African origins" theory smouldered in both popular and scientific forums.

Continued opposite:

caused by HIV-2 have not been reported, they think, is that HIV-2 infection is of a slightly later date than HIV-1 infection. Given time and in the absence of preventive measures, they believe that the HIV-2 epidemic could become just as serious as that of HIV-1.

HIV-2 has now begun to appear in many other parts of the world (see Figure 3.5). The earliest cases in Europe were found in France and Portugal, in patients who had lived in Guinea-Bissau and Angola [22]. It has since been detected in West Germany [23], Denmark, Italy, Norway, Sweden [24] and the United Kingdom [25], as well as in Brazil [26] and the United States [27].

The epidemiology of AIDS

Epidemiology is the study of the incidence and spread of a disease, both internationally and within communities. Understanding how AIDS spreads is important in order to predict where it will occur next,

---

Tempest in a test tube (continued from previous page)

SIV exists, but its origins, like those of HIV-1 and HIV-2, remain unknown, more of a mystery than ever. The most complete genetic analyses of all three viruses indicate that SIV is different enough from both the human viruses that the latter cannot have evolved from it in recent times [32]. HIV-1 and HIV-2 probably evolved from a common ancestor as recently as 40 years ago [33]. But what ancestor? Research to date indicates that this ancestor was probably not SIV.

In other words, the hypothesis which so angered many African commentators — that the global AIDS epidemic started when African green monkeys recently passed a virus to Africans — has been disproved.

Unpublished results by additional groups of researchers confirm a link between SIV and African green monkeys. But this virus did not, it now appears, jump from green monkeys to humans in recent decades [34]. Scientists have been unable to find a relative of SIV in wild monkeys in Asia; investigation of wild monkeys in other parts of the world remains to be done.

Nor have scientists published research into the possibility that the captive monkeys could have caught their virus in other ways. For example, it is theoretically possible that captive monkeys could have contracted a virus from an infected human being, perhaps one of their handlers or keepers. The available evidence cannot rule out the possibility that AIDS viruses passed from humans to primates in other circumstances in some part of the world [35]. Similarly, there is a remote possibility that SIV could be the result of the genetic recombination of viruses found in the captive monkeys' environment.

The true origins of the family of AIDS viruses may be so far in the past that they will never be uncovered. These viruses, which belong to a very small sub-class (the lentiviruses) of the relatively rare group known as the retroviruses, may have been present in the bloodstream of the ancestral creature from whom both Old World primates and human beings are descended. The AIDS virus, or rather its progenitors, may thus be as old, or older, than the human race itself. If this is the case, the important question becomes, why the seemingly sudden appearance of AIDS just decades ago? This is the question on which one research is currently being focused.

and to identify where education and preventive measures would be most effective. So far, the HIV virus seems to have followed three distinct epidemiological patterns. These patterns and the geographic regions in which they are found are described below [36].

Pattern I (homosexual, ivdu, others): introduced or began to spread extensively in mid-1970s or early 1980s; found predominantly in homosexual population (up to 50% of homosexual men in some urban areas are infected) with limited heterosexual transmission (expected to increase). Intravenous drug users (ivdus) account for the second largest proportion of HIV infection (including majority of infection in southern Europe). Transmission via contaminated blood products is not a continuing problem, but tens of thousands were infected by this route before 1985. Perinatal (mother to child) transmission is found primarily among female ivdu, sex partners of ivdu, and women originally from countries where heterosexual spread is common. Infection is distributed in Western Europe, North America, some areas in South America, Australia and New Zealand.

Pattern II (heterosexual, transfusions, others): introduced or began to spread extensively in early to late 1970s; found predominantly in heterosexuals (up to 25% of the 20-40 year old age group in some urban areas and up to 90% of female prostitutes). Homosexual transmission is not a major factor. Transfusion of contaminated blood is a major public health problem. Non-sterile needles and syringes account for an undetermined proportion of infection. Perinatal transmission is a significant problem in areas where 5-15% of women are seropositive. Infection is distributed in Africa, Caribbean, and some areas of South America.

Pattern III (mixed): introduced in early to mid 1980s with spread among persons with multiple sexual partners. Both homosexual and heterosexual transmission has been documented with a current very low prevalence of HIV infection even in persons with multiple partners, such as prostitutes. In some areas ivdu transmission has been recorded. Transmission from contaminated blood is not a significant problem at present, though some infections have occurred in recipients of imported blood or blood products. Perinatal transmission is currently not a problem. Infection distributed in Asia, the Pacific region (minus Australia and New Zealand), the Middle East, Eastern Europe, some rural areas of South America.

Heterosexual spread: where next?

There are strong indications that in a number of countries where the predominant means of transmission of the virus was initially homosexual activity (Pattern I), heterosexual contact (Pattern II) is now playing an increasingly important role. Most of these countries are in Central America and the Caribbean, although there are also areas in United States and European cities where heterosexual transmission is an important factor. In these cities intravenous drug users infected by the virus have infected *their* heterosexual partners, who may in turn later infect others with whom they have sex.

In some parts of Europe (Austria, Italy and Spain are examples) the pattern has changed or is changing from predominantly homosexual contact to transmission through drug use, which in time is likely to lead to greater heterosexual transmission. Elsewhere on the continent heterosexual contact is already a major factor. In Belgium, over 20% of AIDS cases among residents are the result of heterosexual transmission (as are 75% of cases among non-residents, most of whom are from Africa or have lived there). In Portugal, which also has strong African connections, the proportion which falls into this category is 35%, but in Greece, Finland and Switzerland, where the links are more tenuous, the figures are 23%, 17% and 10% respectively [37].

The pattern of transmission is changing rapidly in parts of Latin America and the Caribbean. In Haiti the percentage of men who are believed to have contracted HIV through homosexual activity fell from 56% to 10% between 1983 and 1985, while the percentage of women with AIDS increased from 14% to 36% during the same period [38]. In the 19 small countries which report to the Caribbean Epidemiology Centre (CAREC) the male:female ratio of new cases fell from 6:1 in the second quarter of 1986 to 2.6:1 a year later [39]. In the Dominican Republic and in Honduras over 30% of cases are in women with no history of intravenous drug use.

Although there are no detailed surveys of sexual behaviour in the Caribbean and Latin America, such studies as do exist suggest that many men who are married or who have girlfriends, nevertheless also have frequent sexual relations with other men [40]. One of the leading AIDS experts in Haiti, Dr Jean William Pape, described the situation when his country was a popular destination for homosexual men from the United States on vacation. "It was a prostitution of poverty, of necessity, an economic prostitution. Furthermore, after such intercourse the Haitian man would go to 'cleanse' himself of his 'error' by having relations with a woman, a prostitute or otherwise" [41].

Latin American health officials have voiced their concern that the Haitian pattern could repeat itself in their countries. In Brazil and Mexico, 23% of cases are in men identified as bisexual, a proportion which rises to 40% in Ecuador [42]. In Chile and Venezuela heterosexual contact accounts for 11-12% of cases, while in the French *départements* of French Guiana, Guadeloupe and Martinique the heterosexual pattern has been the norm since the beginning of the epidemic. There has been much debate over the question as to whether widespread heterosexual transmission of HIV will occur in the United States and other Pattern I countries. Early perception of AIDS as a homosexual disease gave way to general fear that it would spread rapidly among the general population as had happened in some central African capitals. In early 1987 the US Secretary of Health and Human Services warned that AIDS was "rapidly spreading" to the wider population and would make the 14th century Black Death in Europe "pale by comparison" [43]. A year later he announced: "We do not expect any explosion into the heterosexual population" [44].

The reasoning behind this shift in attitude is the very slow increase in heterosexual cases recorded by the US Centers for Disease Control in Atlanta. By June 1988 only 4.1% of adult cases in the United States were attributable to heterosexual contact with persons at risk to AIDS, with cases of undetermined origin a further 3.2%. These national figures support the view that AIDS will move only slowly, into heterosexual society at large.

An opposing point of view comes from a report by a team of doctors at the City Hospital in Edinburgh, Scotland, a city where 50% of drug users are seropositive. It points out that nearly one in five of the heterosexual partners of infected drug users pick up the virus, with cases ranging from a 17-year-old girl to a 50-year-old man, neither of whom had other risk factors [45]. The implication is that these partners will go on to infect others. Further evidence of general heterosexual transmission comes from a study carried out in Baltimore, Maryland, where 5.2% of outpatients at an STD (sexually transmitted disease) clinic were found to be seropositive, with half of the women and a third of the men denying high-risk behaviour [46].

Can the opposing points of view be reconciled? Mathematical models of the spread of AIDS are helpful in this respect. British and American epidemiologists who have developed such a model offer the preliminary prediction that in developed countries "the likely scenario for HIV spread is a very slow rise in seropositivity in the general population on a timescale of decades [47].".

The debate over heterosexual AIDS in the United States and Europe is thus less about *whether* it will ever occur, but how far and quickly the virus will diffuse outward from the groups currently at high risk of infection to the population at large. Given the 5-10 year incubation period of AIDS, it is still too early to forecast with certainty the extent to which Pattern II will appear in these countries.

CHAPTER FOUR

WHERE IS AIDS GOING?

The new disease of the 1980s, AIDS has mushroomed from a handful of known cases in 1981 to more than 100,000 officially reported cases affecting 138 countries by the end of June 1988. WHO, governments and agencies participating in the global campaign to check the spread of the AIDS virus acknowledge that the disease poses an unprecedented public health challenge, perhaps the greatest of this century. What can we expect from AIDS? Where will it spread, and how quickly? Can it be controlled, even in seriously-affected countries? Are children at risk from AIDS? And are the so far least-affected countries, mainly in Asia, "safe"?

US blacks and Latinos

The United States was the first country to record its AIDS cases publicly, and there is no doubt that it still has one of the most serious epidemics in the world. But the composition of this epidemic is changing rapidly. Early in 1988, for the first time since AIDS reporting began, the number of new AIDS patients in New York City who are intravenous drug users exceeded the number who are homosexual or bisexual men [1]. In New York City as in the rest of the country, the second wave of AIDS is hitting black and Latino people within whose communities intravenous drug use, poverty, unemployment, discrimination, violent crime, poor health and loss of hope are major problems. Figures published by the US Centers for Disease Control in April 1988 show that for the first time, new cases of AIDS among blacks and Latinos outnumbered those among whites on a nationwide basis.

Among white adults in the United States, the incidence of AIDS cases is 189 per million population; for blacks it is 578 per million; and for Latinos it is 564 per million. Other ethnic minorities in the United States, by contrast, to date appear less affected than whites by HIV infection and AIDS: the remaining population, which includes Asian Americans and Native Americans, has only 74 adult cases per million [2].

However, minority organisations in the United States (and also in Canada) believe that for Native Americans the official figures give a false picture [3]. In most US states and in Canada Native Americans are often classified as Caucasian (white) if they are of mixed native and white parentage or if they do not have "treaty" status. Native Americans with treaty status are those who have documentary proof that they are entitled to live on the "reservations" which are defined by various treaties between the Indian nations and the government of the United States or of Canada. People of Native American descent who do not have "treaty" status, who are of mixed race, or who live off the reservations in towns and cities, may appear in the health statistics as white.

Yet it is precisely those Native Americans likely to be classed as white whom one would expect to be most at risk from AIDS, for they share with many urban blacks and Latinos the same social dislocation, discrimination and low economic status which makes them especially vulnerable to HIV and which cause other indications of underpriviledge such as family breakdown, teenage pregnancy, alcoholism, poor health and intravenous drug abuse. There are some indications, although not yet published and documented, that this vulnerability is causing a higher rate of AIDS and HIV among Native Americans than is indicated by the official figures.

Figure 4.1 In the United States, the proportion of new adult AIDS cases among homosexual men and white adults is falling, while the proportion of black and Latino adults, and of all adult women is rising. Source: US Centers for Disease Control.

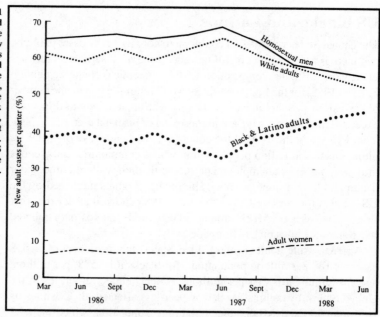

The figures given above mean that a black or Latino person in the United States is three times more likely to have AIDS than a white. And while the rate at which new cases of AIDS are being reported in white adults, and among homosexual men, is slowing a little, the reporting rate for black and Latino adults is accelerating (see Figure 4.1).

Women of colour in the United States are even more vulnerable than men. Black and Latino women account for 71% of all women with

AIDS. A black woman is 13 times more likely to have AIDS than her white counterpart; a Latino woman is nine times more likely [4]. Among blacks and Latinos, heterosexual spread linked to intravenous drug use is undeniably a major factor. Among whites with AIDS, only about 1% are thought to have contracted the virus through heterosexual contact. For Latinos the comparable figure is 4%, and for blacks it is 11%.

'The evolution of AIDS in the USA is a warning to the rest of the world'

By 1991, the United States Public Health Service expects to have a total of 279,000 cases of AIDS. If present trends continue, at least 108,000 of these will be among New York blacks and Latinos, most of them living in low income inner city areas.

Although the most reliable statistics come from New York, other big US cities have similar problems. During 1985/6, testing of blood donors in Atlanta, Baltimore and Los Angeles showed blacks to be over 15 times more likely to carry HIV than whites, with Latinos four times more likely [5]. Nationwide, the picture is similar; blood surveys of military volunteers show that blacks are four times, and Latinos two times, more likely than whites to carry the AIDS virus [6].

The evolution of AIDS in the United States is a warning to the rest of the world. The emerging lesson — that AIDS can take hold in communities made doubly vulnerable by their socio-economic disadvantage and by their lack of information — is a sobering one. This country, one of the world's richest, failed to protect its least powerful citizens from HIV infection, with the result that its minority groups are facing a full-scale epidemic. Throughout the world, wherever such vulnerable communities exist, the threat of an explosion of HIV infection also exists.

AIDS and infants

The spread of HIV in countries where heterosexual transmission is prevalent (see Chapter Three) brings with it an inevitable and dreaded consequence: the birth to HIV-infected mothers of infants who are also infected, and for whom there is little if any hope of survival. Globally, infant AIDS is still in its early days, with the numbers of infected babies that will be born over the next few years likely to rise steeply, in parallel with the fast-growing infection by HIV of young adult women.

In populations where HIV infection is mainly heterosexually transmitted, a substantial proportion of women of childbearing age may now be infected with the virus. An estimated 2-15% of pregnant women in some areas of Central and East Africa are seropositive, and seroprevalence rates of up to 3% have been reported from West Africa [7]. In Europe and the United States, women using intravenous drugs are the primary source of infant infection with HIV [8].

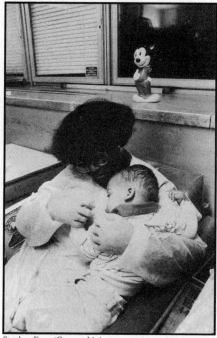

Stephen Ferry/Gamma Liaison

Limited studies from North America and Europe have documented HIV infection in 30-65% of infants of HIV seropositive mothers [9]. Currently, several large studies of perinatal transmission are under way in Africa. In Nairobi, antibody to HIV was detected in 51% of infants born to virus infected mothers. Similarly, 46% of 600 infants of infected mothers in Kinshasa had antibodies to HIV [10].

In New York City a recent blood survey showed that 1.6% of women giving birth in public hospitals were seropositive [11]. In the poor and mainly black neighbourhood of the Bronx, the prevalence of HIV infection was 2.3% [12], a rate similar to that found among mothers in Nairobi, Kenya [13]. In the largely black neighbourhood of Brooklyn, 2% of mothers surveyed in 1987 were seropositive [14]. In the US state of Massachusetts, similar research revealed that in inner city hospitals 0.8% of ante-natal women were seropositive, three times the rate found in more affluent suburban centres [15].

Researchers predict that in the United States up to 4,800 HIV-infected children will be born in 1988, a total expected to rise as more women become infected. As these figures indicate, even where the prevalence of HIV infection among women of child-bearing age is less than 5%, the number of AIDS babies being born is large.

In other parts of the world, for example in Central African cities where the rate of female seropositivity is much higher, the tragedy of infant AIDS increases proportionately. In Rwanda in 1987, 35% of AIDS cases were in children [16], while Zambian health officials suspected that several thousand AIDS babies would be born to Zambian mothers in the same year [17].

The choices for a woman infected with HIV are terrible. The chances are as high as 1 in 2 that her baby will be born carrying the virus, and probably doomed to die of AIDS within two years. Where it is available, many women may opt for a medical termination of the pregnancy. But in many cultures a woman's status, and often her material livelihood, depends on bearing children. In these cultures abortion may be unavailable or illegal. Where, as in much of Africa, infant mortality rates are already so high that women expect up to half their infants to die before the age of five, the 50% risk of delivering an HIV-infected baby may not seem so bad.

'other STDs make it easier for the HIV virus'

Some doctors have suggested, though confirmation is lacking, that pregnancy in a seropositive woman, particularly the last three months, may trigger active replication of the virus and quicken the woman's progress toward fatal AIDS [18]. Very little is yet known about the potential adverse health effects of pregnancy for HIV-positive women, but the possibility that pregnancy could trigger AIDS in the mother has brought suggestions that such women should be advised to consider sterilisation to prevent future pregnancies. This again is a choice which would be ruled out in many cultures.

What will happen to women of such cultural backgrounds when their HIV infection becomes known to family members? Marked with the stigma of being mothers of potential HIV-infected babies, they may be rejected by their husbands and socially ostracised. Cut off from their normal means of economic support, many could be forced into various forms of prostitution in order to survive. Much more research, both on the medical and the social and cultural aspects of AIDS among women and children, is urgently needed.

AIDS follows STDs

People who contract HIV very often have a history of repeated infection with other sexually-transmitted diseases. Homosexual men writing about the AIDS epidemic in their communities in New York and San Francisco have recorded how casually many gay men in the late 1970s regarded their prodigious numbers of sexual partners and their repeated bouts of all manner of STDs [19].

A high level of STDs is clearly related to a high rate of sexual partner change, and frequent sexual partner change has undoubtedly played a role in the AIDS epidemics in Africa and the rest of the Third World, just as it did in encouraging the spread of AIDS among US and European homosexuals. But this is not the whole story in either case. Having certain other STDs makes it easier for the HIV virus to be transferred from one partner to the other during sex.

North American epidemiologists have estimated the risk of contracting HIV in a single act of unprotected heterosexual intercourse with a carrier at less than 1% [20]. Epidemiological studies in Africa [21] and the United States [22] suggest that certain other STDs can make it easier to become infected with the AIDS virus. There are two probable reasons for this. First, many STDs cause ulcers or other sores on the genitals of both men and women; these sores make it easier for the HIV virus to leave one bloodstream and enter the other. Second, when an individual has another sexually transmitted infection, the body sends lymphocytes (the white blood cells which fight disease organisms) to the genital region — and HIV attacks and then lives in these cells.

This increased efficiency of HIV transmission in the presence of other STDs seems to occur regardless of the sex of the partners [23]. For homosexual men, the risk incurred appears to be increased if they engage in unprotected anal intercourse (ie: without using a strong condom). Certain cells found in the lining of the rectum are highly susceptible to infection by HIV [24]. Cells found in the lining of the cervix (the narrow lower end of the female uterus) may also be highly susceptible [25], perhaps becoming infected by semen containing HIV. In Africa, recent research suggests that two STDs (genital ulcer disease and chlamydia trachomatis infection) do indeed play a role in the transmission of HIV independent of the frequency of partner change [26].

Genital ulcer disease and infection by HIV are frequently found in individuals with many sexual partners. It is therefore extremely difficult to show which came first: multiple partners leading to genital ulcers and subsequently infection with HIV, or infection with both genital ulcers and HIV as a result of multiple partners. Recent studies have sought to untangle these factors and their results have important implications.

Women infected with genital ulcer disease or chlamydia, both of which damage the genital membranes are, according to a study carried out in Nairobi, Kenya, much more likely to contract HIV during sexual intercourse with an infected partner than are women without such ulcers [27]. In a group of women studied in Harare, Zimbabwe, the risk of catching HIV tripled for those with a history of genital ulcer disease [28].

Genital ulcers are themselves a result of such sexual infections as herpes, syphilis and chancroid and are therefore common in many countries where STDs are under-treated or badly controlled. Up to one in three people in some groups in Africa have had genital ulcers, which are more visible and thus easier to detect in men than in women. A team of Kenyan and Canadian researchers has published evidence to show that a woman with genital ulcers is four times as likely to contract the AIDS virus from an HIV-infected partner than a women without ulcers [29].

According to one of these researchers, "genital ulcer disease not only makes a woman more susceptible to acquiring the AIDS virus, it also probably makes her more infectious for her sexual partner" [30]. Another of the scientists comments that "in patients who already have the AIDS virus, immune deficiency can predispose them to picking up infections which cause genital ulcers" [31].

In men, genital ulcers can provide an entry point for the passage of the virus from female to male. One African study found that men who had had sex with a woman with genital ulcers had a 5-10% chance of contracting HIV from a single sexual exposure [32]. By contrast, studies of couples where one partner is HIV-positive as a result of blood tranfusion show that for the uninfected partner the risk of acquiring the AIDS virus is 7-23% over a period of years [33].

'since STDs are regarded as shameful, their control is sometimes ignored '

As with other infectious diseases, the problem of controlling STDs is greatest in Third World regions. Successful programmes require that anyone contracting a sexual infection has access to treatment and counselling, and that information about STDs and how they are transmitted is widely available. Control programmes absorb resources, both financial and human, which many developing countries would rather allocate to other serious health campaigns. And since STDs are widely regarded as shameful, their control is sometimes simply ignored in the hope that the problem will go away.

Long before AIDS was heard of, specialists in STDs were arguing that these infections constituted an excessive drain on health resources, especially in Africa and parts of Asia [34]. In the last two decades STDs have been many times more common in some regions of the Third World, both urban and rural, than in North America and Western Europe [35].

"The general impression of many practising physicians", writes one group of African doctors, "is that the STDs, particularly gonorrhoea, may have reached endemic proportions in the urban areas of tropical Africa, with increasing spread to the rural areas [36]".. So common is gonorrhoea among some ethnic groups, African doctors have written, that its symptoms are sometimes regarded as a sign of sexual awakening or potency [37].

"It is obvious", according to Dr A. O. Osoba, a Nigerian STD expert, "that STDs in Africa constitute a major public health problem" [38]. But while in some African regions the problem is especially acute, African countries are not alone in facing serious STD epidemics. High rates of sexual infections are found in many parts of the developing world. The World Health Organization ranks STDs among the Third World's most pressing health problems: malaria, diarrhoeal disease, malnutrition and tuberculosis [39].

Directly comparable data, from which an accurate statistical picture of the relative seriousness of STDs in various developing countries can be built up, is non-existent. However, some comparisons can be made, and they show that STD "hot spots" are dotted around the world with most, though by no means all, of the dots falling in developing countries.

'Bangkok **The drug connection**

showed an   Heroin and other drug users frequently inject directly into their veins —
upsurge of   and share dirty needles. This is another major pathway for spreading
HIV in   AIDS. So far in the United States, most of the heterosexually-infected
drug users'   people with AIDS appear to have been black or Latino women who
were the partners of ivdus (intravenous drug users). Sixty per cent
of heroin addicts in New York City are thought to be HIV-infected,
and officials predict that 100,000 US ivdus will develop AIDS by 1991.
Most of the children in the United States who have developed AIDS
after being infected at birth are the children of black or Latino drug users.

Elsewhere in the world HIV infection amongst drug users has also
risen dramatically. In Europe drug use was responsible for 19.6% of all
AIDS cases registered by December 1987 [40], up from 6.7% in
September 1985 [41]. Intravenous drug use is the major cause of
transmission in Italy and Spain, accounting for 64% and 53% of cases
respectively, while in Austria, Ireland and Yugoslavia more than 20%
of cases are in drug users. In Dublin, Edinburgh, Madrid and Milan,
up to 50% of ivdus have AIDS or HIV infection and these cities have
served as foci for outward spread of the infection. The Italian data are
particularly alarming because syringes are freely available in that
country.

In Bermuda over 60% of AIDS cases are in drug users, but as yet this
risk behaviour has not been a major factor elsewhere in the Caribbean.
In Brazil and Chile drug use accounts for 5-6% of cases, while in
Argentina up to 60% of one group of users were discovered to be
carrying the AIDS virus. Although contaminated needles for medical
or quasi-medical purposes are believed to have led to infection in
Africa, intravenous drug use is almost unknown.

In Hong Kong, a wide-ranging narcotics treatment programme has so
far kept infection amongst drug users to zero, but there are ominous
signs elsewhere in the region. Fewer than 1% of cases in Australia by
mid-1987 were in drug users, but one report has suggested that almost
1% of the whole population were at least casual intravenous drug
users, with needles being shared by 60% of drug users [42].

The most alarming figures, however, come from Bangkok in
Thailand, where a recent government report showed an upsurge of HIV
infection in drug users seeking treatment — from 1% in 1987 to 16%
in 1988. A major factor in this increase has been the change by many
drug users in South-East Asia from inhaling opium derivatives to
injecting them. The Thai experience should serve as a warning, but if
action is not taken it may presage an epidemic in those neighbouring
countries where intravenous drug use is common.

Were will AIDS go next?

Just how extensive is AIDS likely to become? Whom will it affect? Can it be stopped? What measures are needed? No one knows the answer to these questions, and even among medical and other experts opinions vary. Predictions based on these opinions fall into three categories or "scenarios" — the doomsday scenario, the business-as-usual scenario and the containment scenario.

The doomsday scenario

'doomsday advocates see AIDS as a threat to the very existence of the human race'

The doomsday scenario assumes a combination of least likely outcomes: that AIDS education will not work, that everyone who contracts the virus will die and that no effective treatment or vaccine will be discovered. Advocates of this view see AIDS as a threat to the very existence of the human race, and, usually, to their particular national, religious or racial group. Those putting forward doomsday predictions sometimes hold extremist political views or belong to fundamentalist religious sects, though their ranks include a number of scientists from various disciplines. Examples of such use made of doomsday arguments, and the reasons why they can jeopardise AIDS prevention, are given in Chapter Nine.

Doomsday theorists have predicted that AIDS will result in the massive depopulation of heavily affected areas, especially in Central Africa. Such forecasts have sometimes been accompanied by the assertion that the epidemic has progressed to such an extent in these areas that they might as well be abandoned by the rest of the world [43]. Only the most stringent action including mass testing for antibodies to HIV, compulsory HIV test-result cards, quarantine of those found positive, and suppression of homosexuality will, argue the voices of doom, avert a total disaster.

The issue of declining population due to AIDS is one of extreme political sensitivity. From the outset it is important to state that adequate scientific data on which to base firm forecasts of population decline are not at present available. African officials have protested that such forecasts made about their countries are pure guesswork and damaging to their economies and national prestige. The "guesstimates", they say, are largely based on extrapolations from urban seroprevalence statistics. But most African people live in rural areas, the officials explain, and rates of HIV infection in the countryside are very low.

Is AIDS likely to depress population growth rates in hardest-hit countries? There are good reasons for seeking scientific answers to this question: the level of resources invested now in AIDS prevention, and all medium and long term social and economic planning by

'What will happen when people get tired of hearing about AIDS?' governments, are affected by assumptions about the likely impact of AIDS on future population levels.

At present the level of uncertainty attached to population forecasts vis-a-vis AIDS is great. One method of imposing some precision is to attempt to quantify the variables involved, including the level of uncertainty, by means of a computer-based mathematical model. British researchers working with Panos have done this, and published very preliminary results. The results show that under certain conditions AIDS has greater potential to depress population growth rates than historically important epidemics such as smallpox and bubonic plague [44]. The difference between AIDS and plague, however, is that whereas plague spreads rapidly, killing the majority of its victims within weeks or months of the first infection, it takes many years or even decades for the full impact of AIDS mortality to be felt.

According to the British computer model — and the researchers stress that computer models generate results which are only as solid as the data which is fed into them — the unchecked spread of AIDS in some countries where HIV prevalence among urban adults have reached double figures could lead to the onset of population decline within a few decades [45]. But this computer result does *not* affirm the dire predictions of the doomsday theorists, for two reasons.

First, even in the worst-affected countries, population decline due to AIDS is not happening now, and will not occur for at least 20, and possibly as many as 70, years. The chief variable affecting the future death toll from AIDS is the success of AIDS education and prevention programmes implemented from now on. Second, the model's results are based on data and assumptions which may change as more is learned about AIDS. Such results can be usefully employed to inform policy decisions, but only if it is recognised that they are projections, not statements of fact. Unfortunately, this is a distinction which proponents of doomsday scenarios usually ignore.

The business-as-usual scenario

Business-as-usual accurately describes the response of many governments to the AIDS crisis: a mixture of denial, indecision and procrastination. Proponents of this scenario do not disagree that the global mobilisation has thus far been very impressive, but they suspect that such an unusual degree of co-operation is unlikely to persist. What will happen when people get tired of hearing about AIDS, they ask, as has happened on so many other issues of global importance?

Whereas containment advocates (see below) keep their eyes on the future, business-as-usual theorists tend to look to the past. What they see makes them more pessimistic. Syphilis, an STD once feared as much as AIDS, has not been brought under consistent control even *after* the advent of an effective treatment (penicillin). STD control in general waxes and wanes according to public commitment and political will, and, business-as-usual theorists suggest, there is little reason to believe that AIDS control will be any more effective [46].

Another major avenue for the spread of HIV — intravenous drug use — draws similarly pessimistic forecasts for AIDS control. In the United Kingdom, 50% of the drug-takers in one city, Edinburgh, are now carrying HIV, while in a comparable city, Liverpool, seropositivity is negligible. Among reasons cited for this difference are the existence of comprehensive narcotics treatment programmes and easy access to sterile needles in Liverpool, neither of which is available in Edinburgh. Similar differences exist between New York, where 50% seropositivity amongst drug users was reached by 1986 [47], and San Francisco, where the equivalent rate had not risen above 10%-15% by 1987 [48]. Keeping infection rates low seems to be a function of an extensive drugs treatment programme involving the recruitment of ex-addicts as outreach workers, the distribution of free condoms, syringes and bleach (to sterilise needles), and alternative means of drug maintenance or withdrawal. For both political and financial reasons, very few communities are able to offer such a wide range of facilities.

Moreover, say business-as-usual theorists, even if a vaccine or cure is developed, there is no compelling reason to believe that it will be made available to all who need it as a matter of course. Effective treatments, adequate education, counselling and funding may not reach those who need them. The issue is not merely the development of treatments or vaccines, but the efficiency, fairness and consistency with which they are deployed [49].

If the business-as-usual scenario turns out to be correct, AIDS is likely to take root in the most vulnerable and least vigilant groups. Those groups most able to protect themselves, through AIDS education and other measures, will be able to escape the worst ravages of the pandemic. Business-as-usual is a prescription for a world divided by AIDS, and in which the momentum of the pandemic is slowed but not halted, and the lives to be sacrificed are taken from the ranks of the socially and economically disadvantaged.

The containment scenario

Spearheaded by WHO and several committed governments and agencies, an international drive to curb the spread of AIDS was launched in February 1987. The global programme of action being co-ordinated by WHO is described in Chapter Eight. This programme is based on the "containment" scenario: that even in the absence of a vaccine

'Scientists already know more about HIV than about almost any other disease'

against the virus, AIDS can be contained through concerted application of sound public health principles, including both medical and health education measures.Those engaged in the international battle list a number of reasons why their optimism is justified:

● Scientists already know more about HIV than they do about almost any other disease organism.

● AIDS is a global threat, and has evoked unprecedented global co-operation in response.

● The centuries-old scourge of smallpox was eliminate from the world by just such international co-ordination, and other global drives, such as that to immunise the world's children, are meeting with success: an encouraging precedent.

● Some of the avenues by which HIV is spread, such as through blood transfusions, are being cut off in country after country.

● Other avenues, such as the medical use of unsterile needles and syringes, can and will be stopped.

● Condoms offer a degree of protection against HIV infection. and condom sales are increasing in many regions of the world.

● In North America and Europe at least, a widespread epidemic of AIDS among heterosexuals does not seem to be taking off, and may never occur. Widespread AIDS among heterosexuals may be confined to some African and Latin American states.

● In at least one of the Central African cities most affected by AIDS, rates of infection could be levelling off, claim one set of researchers [50] .

● Conservative rural areas of the world may see little growth in HIV infection, as one study of the Equateur province of Zaire has suggested [51] .

● AIDS education can work, as the slowed growth of HIV and other STD infection in homosexual communities in the United States and Europe shows. It is the single most important weapon against AIDS that we possess.

Global AIDS control will work, those who believe in the containment scenario argue.   An indication of its gathering momentum is the AIDS "glasnost" — a new willingness to confront and discuss AIDS on the part of governments which formerly refused to admit the problem — which was demonstrated by the gathering of over 100 health ministers in London during January 1988. Here, in several cases for the first time, health ministers talked about AIDS in their countries with unusual candour.

According to Dr Jonathan Mann, director of WHO's global programme on AIDS, the health ministers' summit "marked a watershed" in the international mobilisation against AIDS. The summit made clearer than ever before that no country anywhere in the world is immune from HIV; that the growth of AIDS cannot be stopped in any one country without being stopped in all countries; and that the best way to stop it is through the open sharing of experience.

'the best we can hope for is to slow down the epidemic'

Containment theorists hope that they can "hold the line" against the AIDS virus, preventing the development of full-scale epidemics in countries where they do not yet exist, until such time as a vaccine against HIV or a cure for AIDS is found and made available.

We can't stop AIDS yet

Of these three scenarios, containment is the most hopeful. Time will tell whether containment is an unduly optimist prospect, or whether the determination of governments and communities will slacken, allowing business-as-usual to take over, and opening the door to some of the more pessimistic doomsday predictions.

But what is clear is that there is at present no more optimistic outcome than containment. Talk of "stopping" AIDS is at present unrealistic. It summons images of the elimination of AIDS from the world in the way smallpox has been eliminated, something which is not yet possible. Until medical science develops effective and cheap vaccines and therapies for AIDS, or until the great majority of humankind adopts complete chastity, neither of which seems likely in the next decade, HIV will continue to spread.

Even if a vaccine were developed tomorrow and every human on the planet were immunised the day after, the number of new cases of AIDS would continue to grow for at least five years as a result of the large number of people already infected.

We can — and must — fight the AIDS epidemic, and we know how to do so. But the medical tools to eliminate AIDS have not yet been developed, and may never be available. Unless or until they are, the best we can hope for is to steadily slow down the growth of the epidemic.

CHAPTER FIVE

PREVENTION MEANS SELF-PROTECTION

So far, education is the best AIDS medicine we have. Spread it around," says an AIDS worker in Brazil.

Until a vaccine is developed, preventing the further spread of the HIV virus can be done only by preventing transmission. There are some actions which only governments or health authorities can take — and they depend on adequate funds and medical staff:

- Screening blood supplies, to remove blood contaminated with the HIV virus.
- Supplying vaccination programmes with sterilising facilities for reusable syringes or, alternatively, with once-only syringes.
- Ensuring that every citizen, including the young, receives information on HIV and on how it is spread.
- Ensuring adequate availability of condoms.
- Making free, confidential HIV testing and counselling available.
- Supplying treatment, clean needles and/or bleach (to sterilise needles) to intravenous drug users.
- Ensuring that people with HIV or AIDS, or those who think they might be at risk, are protected from discrimination so that they feel free to seek the help they need.

All these actions depend heavily on governments, but most prevention hinges mainly on the responsible actions of the individual. He and she can adopt safer sex practices; avoid those few other activities which can transmit the infection; and influence family, friends and colleagues to do likewise.

What is safer sex?

"Unless it is possible for you to know with absolute certainty that neither you nor your sexual partner is carrying the AIDS virus, you must use protective behaviour. Absolute certainty means not only that you and your partner have had a faithful monogamous sexual relationship for at least five years, but that neither you nor your partner has used illegal intravenous drugs," wrote the US Surgeon-General in November 1986. Though sober in the extreme, this advice is good all over the world, especially where the AIDS virus is already present.

The key to personal action against AIDS is safer sex. Just what forms of sex are safe, and unsafe? As the risks of various methods of transmission are studied more carefully, advice on safer sex is becoming clearer and more specific.

HIV can be present in the semen and vaginal fluids of HIV- positive people. The most dangerous form of sexual activity is, without any doubt, penetrative sex: sex in which the man's penis enters the vagina or the anus (rectum) of a woman or the anus of another man. It is likely that the AIDS virus can be passed from penis to rectum and vagina or vice versa in the absence of tears in the genital tissues or bleeding, especially when genital ulcers are present. There is strong scientific evidence that correct use of a condom can reduce the risk enormously.

There is still some uncertainty about the degree of risk involved in oral sex (in which the mouth comes into contact with semen or vaginal secretions); such activity is best avoided. Semen should never be swallowed, and a male should not ejaculate in his partner's mouth. This is especially important where either partner has sores on the sex organs or bleeding or sores in the mouth.

HIV has been detected in saliva, but there is no evidence that kissing can transmit the virus. So far as is known, deep kissing (where the tongue enters another person's mouth) is not a risky activity. But some education campaigns have cautiously listed deep kissing as only "possibly safe", and advised people that for complete safety they should limit themselves to "dry kissing" on the lips or body only.

Forms of sex which can involve bleeding (bondage, sado-masochism or intercourse during menstruation etc) are probably high-risk activities.

Because safe sex advice has often been seen as negative and therefore unlikely to change people's behaviour, some campaigns have focused on more positive aspects. Danish television slots have emphasised "Sex is beautiful" while promoting use of the condom. In Kenya and Uganda the slogan "Love carefully" does not discourage lovemaking, but suggests that partners in the act care for one another by the responsible use of condoms. In Britain the voluntary organisation the Terrence Higgins Trust has encouraged people to place less emphasis on intercourse and more on the pleasures of various forms of massage, embracing and safe sex games.

Condoms work

Condoms (rubber sheaths) are a vital component of safe sex and a key element in AIDS education and prevention.

Who uses condoms? Before the dangers of AIDS were recognised, 27% of all condom users were in Japan (where the contraceptive pill is

'street sellers
of condoms say
AIDS has done
wonders for
their business'

rare), 38% in the rest of the developed world, and 18% in China. Latin America and the Caribbean accounted for only 3% of world condom use and Africa and the Middle East only 1% [1].

Condoms have not always been easy to obtain in the Third World, or in the countries of Eastern Europe. When they are available, they have often been old and defective. Cultural, religious and social attitudes have often prevented men using them. In many parts of Africa they have been seen as the white man's means of keeping black population numbers down. In Brazil and other countries they have been associated with disease; producing one before intercourse implies that one's partner is unclean. In Bangladesh condoms were not used because of traditional beliefs — for example "semen is a necessary health tonic for women" and "condoms can cause impotence" [2]. Worldwide the Roman Catholic church objects to their function as contraceptives, although in some countries, eg: Uganda and Brazil, it has recognised their use in the fight against AIDS.

Laboratory tests have demonstrated that the AIDS virus does not penetrate rubber latex condoms [3]. Studies of female prostitutes in Zaire [4] and heterosexual couples in Florida [5] have shown significantly lower rates of seropositivity in individuals who insist on condom use. Homosexual men who practise safer sex, including the use of condoms, are also less likely to be infected [6].

Until very recently, the use of condoms in North America and Western Europe had declined as other means of contraception, particularly the pill, were adopted. However, following the use of condoms by homosexual men for anal intercourse, there has been a rapid increase in condom sales for heterosexual use. One of the world's largest manufacturers, London International Group, announced a 40% increase in shipments in 1987 [7], while sales in the United States rose from 182 million in 1980 to 406 million in 1987 [8]. In West Germany sales rose 90% between February and May 1987; in Australia they were up 35% in the same period [9]; following the repeal of laws banning the advertising of condoms in France, sales rose 38% [10].

According to one of the world's major distributors, the International Planned Parenthood Federation (IPPF), it is too early to say that condom use is rising dramatically as a result of AIDS. There are, however, reports of an increase in demand in many places. In 1988 Bem-Fam, the Brazilian family planning association, has supplemented its annual order of 6 million from IPPF with 12 million from USAID (see below) [11]. Trinidad's supply from the same source has risen by 50% in 1988 [12]. In Bogotá, Colombia, street sellers of condoms say AIDS has done wonders for their business [13]. In half a dozen African countries, such as Nigeria and Tanzania, demand has risen significantly [14] and Panos has received many undocumented reports that the street price of condoms has risen as a result.

Many family planning organisations and health clinics worldwide distribute condoms free. The biggest supplier to the Third World is USAID, the overseas funding agency of the United States Government, which was scheduled to purchase and distribute 750 million sheaths worldwide in 1987: enough to supply every married couple in a country the size of Zaire for 12 months. In the same year British businessman Richard Branson, founder of the Virgin group of companies, entered the market with condoms offered to the public at cut-price and to health clinics at cost (6 US cents), with profits going to AIDS charities. In early 1988 he was reportedly invited to supply the Soviet Union with condoms to supplement the limited and often poor quality products currently available.

A form of condom was used by the ancient Egyptians, and varieties have been found the world over for a number of centuries. Recently, however, there has been a novel development, the *female* condom. Developed in Denmark and tested in Britain, it is scheduled to go into production towards the end of 1988. Inserted like a diaphragm or tampon, it is held in place by an outer ring. In trials both men and women said that they found it preferable to the male condom. Initial predictions were that they would reach 10% of the US condom market of 4 billion units a year [15]. Although there are as yet no public plans to distribute it elsewhere, the female condom could have a major role to play in contraception and disease prevention in future years.

Education: signs of success

In many countries information produced and distributed by organisations of homosexual men has been the best and until recently the only source of information on AIDS. Two of the oldest and best-known of these organisations are the Gay Men's Health Crisis (GMHC) in New York (founded in 1982), and the Terrence Higgins Trust in London (founded in 1983) [16]. Others have followed, including Aides in France, the Bobby Goldsmith Foundation in Australia and AIDS Vancouver in Canada.

Their experience of raising awareness about the AIDS virus is still probably the most extensive available. Although their messages have been aimed predominantly at homosexual men, their methods — sticking to the facts, using blunt everyday language, emphasising individual responsibility and self-respect, and involving group members in all aspects of the prevention programme — are applicable elsewhere. Evidence of how communities threatened by AIDS can mobilise their resources also comes from homosexual

'volunteers in organisations.   In the financial year 1985-86, volunteers in San
San Francisco Francisco gave 130,000 person-hours of unpaid time, answered over
gave 130,000 30,000 telephone enquiries, and distributed over 240,000 leaflets on
hours of unpaid AIDS prevention. Home-based care was provided to 165 patients at an
time' average cost of US$94 a day, greatly reducing hospital costs [17]. In
1987 GMHC raised half of its US$3.6 million budget from voluntary
sources, enabling it to employ over 50 paid staff.

What effect has this type of activity had on sexual behaviour among
homosexual men? Studies in San Francisco, New York, Los Angeles,
Denver and Pittsburgh, and similar research in Canada, the United
Kingdom and France, have shown that the sexual behaviour of
homosexual men has indeed been changing. The rate of reporting of
new   HIV infections and of some other STDs   has   slowed
dramatically.

In San Francisco, the annual rate at which homosexual men were
becoming HIV-positive fell from 17% in 1982-84 to 4% in 1984-85,
while the incidence of rectal gonorrhoea (an STD found almost
exclusively among homosexual men) has fallen by 71% between 1983
and the end of 1985. In London (UK) in mid-1986, 77% of
homosexual men questioned claimed to follow "safer sex"
guidelines, and 48% said they were having fewer partners than a year
before. The city's incidence of STDs among homosexual men has
fallen, while among heterosexuals it continues to rise.   In the United
States between mid-1987 and mid-1988 the proportion of new cases of
AIDS in homosexual men with no history of drug use has fallen from
69% to 56%.

It is not clear how much of this change is the result of education
and how much is a result of the fact that most homosexual men have
seen several friends or acquaintances die of AIDS. But the importance
of education is not in doubt. In a relatively short space of time,
through trial and   error, homosexual men's groups learned how to
select, version and target information about AIDS to best effect in their
own communities. What then, are the conditions under which AIDS
education becomes effective?

AIDS campaigns: pointers and pitfalls

Hundreds, perhaps even thousands of AIDS awareness campaigns are
being put into operation around the world. Some important lessons
are emerging.

*By itself, information increases knowledge but does not change
behaviour.* In several countries governments have run multi-media
mass alert campaigns on AIDS. The results? People know more about

AIDS and how the virus is transmitted, but this in itself seems to have little influence on their behaviour.

In Britain a year after the intensive government campaign under the slogan "Don't Die Of Ignorance", up to 93% of teenagers knew how AIDS was transmitted. But 33-50% of 16-24 year olds — a group at high risk — said that absence of a condom would not prevent them from having intercourse [18].

AIDS educators must understand and confront people's fears. If they fail to do this, they are unlikely to promote

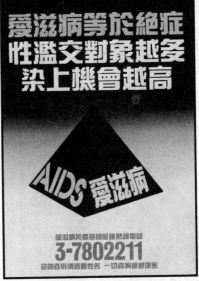

Figure 5.1
Hundreds, perhaps thousands, of AIDS education campaigns are now under way all over the world. This leaflet is from Hong Kong, and is headed "AIDS equals fatal disease". The Chinese ideogram for AIDS means "love disease".

meaningful behaviour changes. In fact, AIDS information which stirs up fears of contagion in the absence of supportive discussion and counselling can be worse than no information at all, increasing irrational behaviour and stigmatisation.

In Japan many people "think that foreigner equals AIDS carrier", according to one AIDS specialist. An opinion survey found that 85% of teachers knew that AIDS could not be contracted from swimming pools or from Western-style toilet seats. But 45% still said they did not like using pools or toilets in places frequented by foreigners [19].

The source of AIDS information must be trusted. People seldom act constructively on the basis of information which is delivered by people or institutions whose motives they suspect. "The first principle", says an AIDS educationist with the New York City public health department, who works with drug users, "is to build trust around you and your team and not to underestimate the people you are trying to reach. You treat a junkie from the streets with the same respect you treat a doctor." [20]

In Washington DC young blacks in the inner city "perceive AIDS as some sort of germ warfare created in government labs to be used against them.... Past failure to deal effectively with other problems, like the war on poverty and the war on drugs ... adds to their disbelief when it comes to government officials telling them that now there is a war on AIDS." [21]

Figure 5.2
Although some
eastern
Mediterranean
countries were
initially slow to
acknowledge the
danger posed by
AIDS, 13 countries
in the region have
established national
AIDS committees.
This leaflet is from
Kuwait.

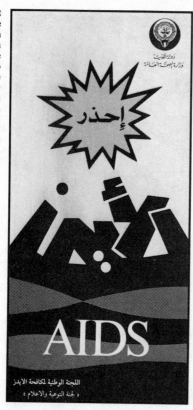

To educate people about AIDS, it is first necessary to overcome denial. Almost every community in the world which has been faced with the problem of AIDS has first reacted by denying the existence of the problem. Sometimes denial takes the form of a feeling of personal invulnerability to AIDS. Until the fact that there is a problem is acknowledged, modifying risk behaviours is not possible.

In Zambia a prostitute who works in Lusaka said: "I contracted other diseases but got cured. There is no incurable disease that I have contracted, and there is a medicine for every disease. The truth about AIDS is that it doesn't exist." [22] In Nigeria a Lagos-based prostitute says: "Although white clients generally pay better than their African counterparts, I will never go to bed with a white man unless he wears a condom. As far as I am concerned, AIDS is a white man's disease." [23]

In New York City in 1986, when outreach workers began to talk to the Latino community about AIDS the response was: "Why are you talking to us about this? It's a disease of whites, of homosexuals and drug addicts. We don't have those kind of people here." [24] In San Francisco "teenagers who were educated about the risks of AIDS developed a sophisticated awareness of its dangers ... but large numbers continued to engage in high risk sex. Young people in particular may understand the educational messages [but] they just don't believe that the disease will strike them." [25]

AIDS information must take account of actual sexual behaviour. "The more experience I have with this epidemic", says a prominent US public health specialist, "the more it becomes apparent that a key and neglected factor is bisexuality" [26]. "

In Brazil "a great many Brazilian men who engage in same-sex interaction don't identify themselves as homosexuals or bisexuals" [27]. Health officials throughout the Latin American region fear that the denial that homosexuality exists presents them with one of the most difficult challenges in raising awareness about the threat of AIDS [28].

In Tanzania "when 35-year-old Lenika Savorek read a poster explaining that to avoid infection with AIDS he should 'have sex with only one faithful partner' he burst into laughter. 'What am I going to do with my other wives?', he asked [29]. "Love carefully", the slogan adopted by the Ugandan campaign, recognises the existence of polygamy in local cultures.

Religion and culture are powerful in shaping attitudes toward AIDS. AIDS information ignores these factors at the cost of failing to get the message across.

In the United States religion can condition responses to the threat of AIDS, and "black Americans, particularly women, frequently cope with psychological difficulties through prayer.... for a miracle" [30]. In California "a recent poll found that almost 40% of fundamentalist Christians believed that AIDS is a punishment from God for the way homosexuals live," and looking after people with AIDS may be "interfering with God's plans" [31]. In parts of Zambia, "when a man dies his male relatives must have sex with his widow. A ward chairperson of the ruling party in Lusaka's Kapwepwe ward has been quoted as saying that it is wrong for anybody to forsake their culture because of AIDS." [32]

AIDS education among women must take account of their social and cultural situations. Studies show that quite often women are more afraid of AIDS than are men, but in many cultures restrictions on their personal autonomy prevents them from taking risk-reducing actions such as insisting that male sexual partners always use condoms. In the United States "a women who initiates discussion about AIDS [in the Latino community] is seen as signalling that she is a loose woman. The feeling is that if she is a good

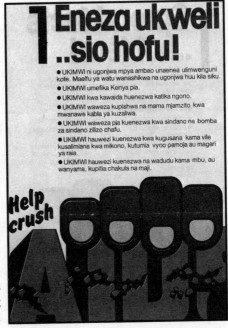

Figure 5.3
AIDS education campaigns are now under way in many languages. "Spread facts not fear! Help crush AIDS!" says this Kenya Red Cross leaflet in Swahili.

The Rwandan campaign

Rwanda is an East African state about the size of Switzerland with a population of 6.8 million. It also has the world's 12th highest number of reported AIDS cases per capita. In 1985 the country embarked on what is so far the best co-ordinated AIDS education campaign in the Third World. Rwanda's campaign is not perfect, but in some respects it is a model of how a small-to-medium sized country can start to inform its entire population about the risks of AIDS.

After surveying adults to find out what they knew and didn't know about AIDS and how it is transmitted, the campaign co-ordinators launched a full-scale publicity effort with a series of radio programmes and the distribution of 35,000 information booklets throughout the country.

Rwanda has the advantage of a well-developed administrative and comunications structure based on units ranging from districts ("prefectures") to sub-districts ("communes") and local groups ("cellules") consisting of 50 families — 700 people each. Over 60% of Rwandans can read, and each local unit is led by a person who is literate. Co-ordinated by the Rwandan Red Cross, which is well-rooted in Rwandan society at all levels, the education programme first targeted the leaders at each administrative level. They were the recipients of the AIDS booklet, and once they had read, discussed and learned it, the country was saturated with shorter and simpler leaflets on AIDS.

On picking up a leaflet, the average Rwandan could then turn to a community leader at each administrative level to ask questions or request further information. Preliminary evaluation of the programme shows that knowledge of AIDS has improved, but it is too early to tell whether changed sexual behaviour will follow [41]. By autumn 1988, the Red Cross plans to have ready a leaflet for distribution to all Rwanda's secondary school students. Before that, however, a manual on AIDS education will be given to teachers, who will be counselled about how to answer student questions on AIDS [42].

Rwanda's concerted programme, led by the Red Cross rather than the national AIDS committee, should soon reach every segment of society. Its success in slowing the spread of the AIDS virus will interest all those involved in AIDS education

woman, she wouldn't know anything about it." [33]. In New York City "inner-city women at high risk of AIDS infection are now well-informed of their risk but few are changing their behaviour.... In large part ... opposition from men was discouraging women from changing their sexual practices." [34] In Tanzania, 28-year-old Daniel is a truck driver who works between Dar es Salaam and Rwanda. "It's like a sock", he says, "and that part of the body is not meant to have socks on" [35].

Summarising the lessons learned thus far, Dr Allan Brandt, a Harvard medical historian and author of a major work on the history of STD control programmes in the United States, says that there is a strong consensus that AIDS education is urgent. But "I don't think we've thought clearly enough about what that means in the long term."

He cautions that those who assume that education programmes should have quick, decisive results have ignored many public health realities. "I think there's considerable evidence that these measures will fail" [36].

Brandt's message is "No single intervention — even an effective vaccine — will adequately address the complexities of the AIDS epidemic [37]." To be effective in changing sexual and other risk behaviours, and to sustain the change over long periods of time, AIDS education must be part of coherent and comprehensive AIDS prevention programmes. There is no *one* answer, and no *universal* approach to AIDS education.

Different peoples, different messages

"I have one and a half tons of information booklets to distribute", said Gabon's health minister, Jean-Pierre Okias, as he set off for London for the 1988 WHO global health ministers' summit [38]. Dr Okias is part of a growing army of educationalists and researchers spreading information about AIDS in Third World communities. The information is turning up in unexpected places. Sit down for a glass of beer in a Latin American beer garden and you may notice a leaflet telling you how condoms can protect you from contracting HIV. If you are a farmer in rural Malawi, you may find that your agricultural extension worker, who normally tells you about fertilisers and pesticides, is counselling you on how to avoid the risk of HIV infection.

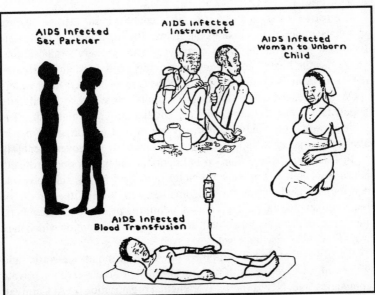

Figure 5.4
AIDS education must use images that relate to the societies they are reaching. This poster comes from a Ugandan teaching kit for secondary schools, and suggests the use of drama, song and puppets to teach about HIV transmission and the need for compassion for people with AIDS.

In Uganda, many rural people are illiterate, and the majority do not have a radio or television. So AIDS education is approached through three principal organisations: through the church, because 92% of the population attend Anglican or Roman Catholic services regularly; through the ruling party's Resistance Committees found in every village; and through schools. Public meetings and political rallies are also used to spread the message, while both major churches have co-operated in a government AIDS education campaign which includes the encouragement of condom use. In the largely Catholic Central African Republic, the church is also informing its members about AIDS: religious comic books used to teach the tenets of the faith now contain references to HIV and AIDS.

AIDS education is already in the health syllabus drawn up by UNICEF for Ugandan primary schools, while teaching on AIDS prevention in secondary schools has already started [39]. In Burundi a conference on AIDS has been held in every school. Students in Sierra Leone wrote a play about AIDS, and the play is now travelling the country, being performed in other schools [40].

In Zambia the students in one school formed an "Anti-AIDS" club. In order to join they pay a small membership fee and promise both to abstain from sex until marriage and to help "protect my relatives and friends by telling them about AIDS". Members get a badge and a club T-shirt with the slogan "AIDS kills, life is precious". The patron, a primary health care doctor, believes it is the first such club in the world and hopes the idea will spread to other schools in Zambia and the rest of the world.

Zimbabwe was one of the first countries in Africa to use nationals rather than outside consultants for its education campaign. In 1987 a team from the army, employers' and workers' organisations, as well as the health, education, community and agricultural sectors, drew up a print and visual campaign in the country's three most widely spoken languages [43]. Here too schools were to be specifically targeted, as were the armed forces, another group at high risk. The project was later shelved, officially because of a shortage of paper, although some reports alleged a change of heart by the government [44].

In Mauritius, where tourism is important for the economy, health educators conduct seminars for hotel managers to consider possible distribution mechanisms for condoms [45]. In Nigeria the union of hotel workers has taken the step of admitting prostitutes as members. Being part of a union allows them access to medical attention which they would not otherwise have [46].

Brazil has distributed pamphlets on AIDS in monthly electric and water bills, as well as with the pay cheques of civil servants, private companies and NGOs (non-governmental organisations). At Carnival,

a time of greater sexual activity, a leaflet in four languages encouraging
the use of condoms was distributed to visitors arriving at airports.
Television spots aimed at people at high risk, particularly at
prostitutes and homosexual men, have been broadcast late at night.

'Maria said yes to all men'

Brazil's government campaign has not been trouble-free.
Television spots have been censored by the Ministry of Health; the
Roman Catholic Church objected to references to condoms; and
cutbacks have been imposed by the country's economic situation.
Because of the country's size and financial difficulties, local initiatives
are more likely to be successful than federal campaigns from
Brasília. Already a homosexual organisation in Salvador is
co-operating with the local family planning organisation, and support
groups for people with AIDS have been set up in Rio de Janeiro and São
Paulo.

The power of pop

Brazil has not been the only country to use television for AIDS
education. In 1987 Britain launched a massive multi-media
campaign designed to alert the public. Pop stars gave warnings about
AIDS on radio, demonstrated the use of condoms on model penises on
television and talked about their attitudes to sex on chat shows. In
Denmark television spots featured children's stories adapted to remind
couples to use condoms, as well as a pop song encouraging people to
protect the one they love. In the Philippines several special episodes of
a popular television soap opera were used to tell viewers about the AIDS
virus and how to avoid it.

Developing countries with a strong pop music tradition have
devised their own ways of using song and pop stars to promote AIDS
education. In Guinea-Bissau in 1987 there were 23 contestants and
a packed stadium for the country's first AIDS song contest. The
winner sang about Maria, the girl with the beautiful body "who said yes
to all men... after one, two, three years, she became so thin". By the end
of the song the audience were all joining in the refrain: "We must be
careful, this is the disease of the century. It has such power." [47].

Why is song so effective? In Guinea-Bissau, where 80% of people
are illiterate, music represents one of the few avenues of
communication with potential to reach the entire population. The radio
network does not cover the whole country, but a catchy pop song with a
message has a good chance of circulating beyond the broadcast net
through portable battery-powered cassette tape decks, especially to
teenagers and young adults, the group most at risk from the AIDS virus.
A similar approach has been adopted in Kenya [48].

One of Zaire's best-known singers, Franco, recorded an album with

'*50% of the women now insist their clients use condoms*' the title "Watch out for AIDS". The title song can be heard playing not just in Kinshasa but in record shops in Paris, London and New York, an indication of the international nature of pop music as a medium for AIDS messages.

Prostitutes protect themselves

Prostitution is a worldwide phenomenon, from the high-earning university-educated New York call girl to the illiterate Third Worlder sitting in a bar and wondering where the next meal is coming from. Money is not always the object; many who offer themselves to strangers are looking for marriage or some form of security. They do not see themselves as prostitutes and prefer to call themselves dancers or hospitality workers.

In a number of east and central African cities prostitutes run very high risks of contracting AIDS. In Nairobi, low income female prostitutes cater to the truck drivers who journey from the port of Mombasa into Uganda and beyond.

In 1980, none of the women tested positive for the AIDS virus. In 1983, 53% of them were HIV-positive, and by 1987 the figure had risen to 80% [49].

An AIDS prevention campaign began in 1985. A public health worker spent several months meeting and getting to know the women, and drew about 300 of them to a public meeting held at the end of the year. There, the women themselves decided that they needed to learn how to control and prevent AIDS. They elected a committee of community leaders, who were trained in how to motivate the others to promote condom use. Those women who had the best knowledge of AIDS prevention shared their knowledge with the others. There was group and individual counselling, where the women could discuss their problems and how to overcome them.

A project leader wrote a song to be sung at the public meetings. The project uses role playing and dramatisation with great success to convey the basics of safer sex.

The results have been a remarkable rise in condom use; 50% of the women now say that they insist their clients use condoms all the times and another 40% report occasional use. There has been a significant drop in the rate at which new women are becoming infected with the virus. And the women have been encouraging their clients to use condoms at home, too [50].

The project demonstrates clearly that the message itself may be less important than the way it is conveyed. But the exploitation which often accompanies Third World prostitution can create a feeling of hopelessness that makes AIDS education difficult.

In the Philippines, some of the "hospitality girls" who provide "R&R" (rest and recreation) services for the US military base have already been infected with AIDS. Their "working hours, drugs and lack of intellectual stimulation stagnate their ability to think about their lives", commented a social worker in mid-1987. "Their isolation and lack of control over their own lives instils the belief that they are powerless individuals and can only survive by complying with the demands of the bar owners and customers and/or outsmarting them". Perhaps as a result, AIDS education has so far had little impact among them [51]. Recently, however, a consortium of Filipino women and health NGOs has formed a task force to advise the government on means of informing and counselling those at high risk. One example of a local campaign has been the "AIDS Roadshow": a theatre performance put on by a women's group, which is both popular and accessible.

'The life of a male prostitute is little better'

The life of male prostitutes is often little better. As young as their mid-teens, they sometimes face an even greater risk of contracting HIV than their female counterparts. In 1987 blood surveys of more than 15,000 prostitutes of both sexes in Thailand showed that whereas 0.05% of the women tested seropositive, 2.6% of the men had been infected [52]. AIDS education in the red-light areas of Bangkok and other cities has been sporadic and bureaucratic, but now some of the women from those districts are educating other sex-industry workers and distributing cheap condoms. So far, however, the bulk of activity seems to be directed at women.

Culture counts

Education programmes and messages designed for the industrialised countries are often inappropriate in the Third World; traditional customs and beliefs may be effective vehicles for indigenous campaigns. And tradition can extend beyond education — in Uganda people with AIDS are reporting that local herbal medicines give relief from some symptoms.

Many Aborigines in Australia have a health status similar to that found in Third World countries, with widespread malnutrition, substandard living environment and poor education. In order to reach this population with effective AIDS education, Australian community health workers use established Aborigine health worker networks. Workshops have been trying out and then adapting various messages. It was, for example, discovered in one area that "condom" was not a good word to use for the sheath, because it is similar to the name of a local tree and many Aborigine women thought they could avoid AIDS by eating its fruit. Another key point was to print leaflets in red, yellow and black:

the colours of the Aborigine flag, which identifies the message as one which Aborigines can trust.

Voodoo, a traditional system of religious belief, is an important element of popular culture in Haiti. An AIDS education campaign for the farm workers of Belle Glade, Florida, incorporated elements of voodoo belief into the AIDS messages for Haitian immigrants. "Pamphlets failed here", said one of the leaders of the campaign, "because so many people can't read" [53]. A better approach started with the traditional explanation of disease in voodoo: that illness is caused by a bad spirit or evil spell.

"Many of the Haitian immigrants I talk to are not only illiterate, but living in a situation where they are deprived of accurate information about a lot of things which affect their daily lives. In some ways this results in them having a very simple world view. I ask them what they know about AIDS, and if they relate sickness to evil spirits, I talk to them about AIDS as an extremely mean spirit that tries to trick them, to make them feel well, so that they go out and spread the evil spell among the people they love. And then I follow the voodoo principle by telling them that they can trick the spirit by practising safer sex." [54]

This chapter has barely touched on the thousands of AIDS education initiatives being taken worldwide. Many will not be successful, like the early leaflets for the Latino community in the United States, which were only translations of leaflets directed at English-speaking homosexual men. Some of these leaflets focused on the mother's role in warning her son to take a contraceptive with him when he went out; in the Latino community there is no tradition of mothers talking to their sons about sex and the leaflets therefore had no interest or appeal to the people at whom they were aimed [55]. Many initiatives will succeed in changing people's behaviour only part of the time, like the men in the Dominican Republic who now use condoms for casual sex, but not with their regular partners [56]. Many other initiatives, particularly those aimed at schoolchildren, will take years to prove their success or failure.

What is important, however, is that the initiatives continue and that they involve not just the professional educationalists and medical workers but all those they are aimed at. In the words of Dr Ruhakana Rugunda, a former minister of health in Uganda and one of the world's pioneers in AIDS prevention: "AIDS is not just a doctor's business, or a nurse's business or an expert's business. Everybody, everywhere, is needed to assist in every way to spread the word on AIDS" [57].

CHAPTER SIX

BLAME AND PREJUDICE

A IDS is overwhelmingly a sexually-transmitted disease, although the virus which causes it can also be transferred by contaminated needles, through contaminated blood, and from mother to child before, during and possibly after birth.

To understand how HIV spreads we need to know much more about sexual habits in different countries and communities. However, sex in nearly all human societies is surrounded by taboos. Few people discuss such a sensitive issue without making or implying moral judgments — or feeling that moral judgments are being made about them. And when people from one ethnic group discuss AIDS in another ethnic group, which inevitably involves discussing other people's sexual behaviour, suspicions of racial and ethnic prejudice are easily aroused.

Discussions about AIDS and sexual behaviour have become complicated by racial prejudices, real and perceived. Other key elements of the AIDS debate have a similar capacity for arousing inter-racial tensions. Where did the disease first originate? Are some racial groups more susceptible to it than others? Should countries screen foreign tourists or businessmen or students to prevent the entry of HIV-infected people? What is the role of prostitution in different societies? How many sexual partners do people have, and how does this vary from one community to another?

These issues are all more or less important, and have to be discussed if the AIDS pandemic is to be fought. But all these issues have acquired moral overtones, of which the main one is the question of blame.

The third epidemic

Blaming other people for a problem, as a substitute for tackling the problem itself, is a very human characteristic. Societies are especially liable to blame other people when misfortunes seem inexplicable or outside their control — something that applies particularly to AIDS.

The process of attributing blame does not always require evidence, and tends to focus on people who are not considered 'normal' by the majority, especially on minorities or foreigners. Epidemics of dangerous infections such as plague, smallpox, syphilis or even influenza, have historically prompted social responses based on blaming others for spreading the disease by their "deviant" behaviour. Blaming others may

**Figure 6.1
Police in
Washington DC
— unnecessarily
clad in rubber
gloves — arrest a
PWA (person
with AIDS) at a
protest march
during the 1987
international
conference on
AIDS. Behaviour
of this sort by
official agencies
reinforces the
incorrect view
that AIDS can be
spread by touch,
and encourages
blame rather than
compassion to be
directed at PWAs.**

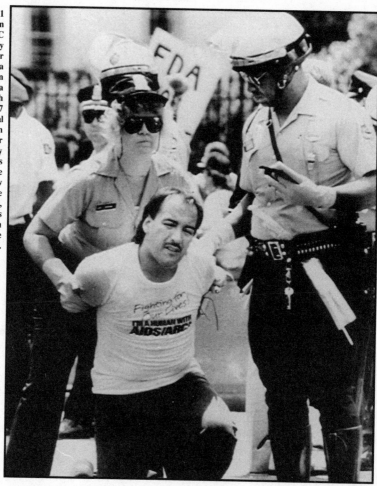

Associated Press

itself be a contagious psychological process, leading on to stigmatisation, scapegoating and persecution [1].

When whole communities blame others for a problem, the results can be traumatic. When the Black Death, an epidemic of bubonic plague, swept across Europe in the 14th century, blame was variously attached to Jews and witches, followed by massacres and burnings of the alleged culprits. And when Hitler blamed Jews, communists, homosexuals, Gypsies and other 'undesirables' for the economic stagnation of Germany in the 1920s, the result was death camps and European war.

Dr Jonathan Mann, who heads the World Health Organization's global programme on AIDS, points out that there are really *three* AIDS epidemics, which are in fact phases in the invasion of a community by the AIDS virus. Each community attacked by AIDS suffers the three phases consecutively.

The first epidemic is one of silent infection by HIV, often completely unnoticed.

The second, after a delay of several years, is the epidemic of the disease AIDS itself, of which more than 100,000 cases had been reported worldwide by the end of June 1988.

The third is the epidemic of social, cultural, economic and political reactions to AIDS, which is also worldwide, and "as central to the global AIDS challenge as the disease itself" [2].

'CDC was defining Haitians as a high-risk group for AIDS'

Pointing to Haiti

Two parts of the developing world, Haiti and Africa, have received widespread publicity as the possible birthplace of AIDS. Haiti, a Caribbean nation whose people are racially of African descent, was singled out first.

In mid-1982, the US Centers for Disease Control (CDC) — the federal public health laboratory — published a new piece of information on the mysterious disease which had already killed nearly 100 US homosexual men, and infected nearly 200 more. In just over a year, said CDC, five US states had reported 34 cases of the new illness in Haitian patients. Thirty of the 34 were men, who denied homosexual activity or drug use. Was this a new clue to the nature of the disease? CDC alerted physicians with Haitian patients to "be aware that opportunistic infections may occur in this population" [3]. Soon, CDC was defining Haitians, along with homosexual and bisexual men, haemophiliacs, and intravenous drug users, as a "high-risk group" for AIDS.

By mid-1983, this view was under attack by Haitian physicians working in the United States. Since Haitians made up only 6% of the 1,220 reported AIDS cases, and any other US ethnic group could have made up a similar or greater percentage of the total, why were Haitians being singled out, the Haitian doctors asked [4]?

Haitian men, they said, were normally reluctant to admit to homosexual activity or to intravenous drug use. The problem was not the lack of other risk factors, but the unfamiliarity of non-Haitian US researchers with Haitian attitudes towards these matters. More sensitive interviewing of patients could have revealed the true risk factors involved, according to the Haitian doctors.

The categorisation of Haitians, like homosexuals and drug addicts, in a separate "risk group" was, says Dr Jean Pape, one of Haiti's leading AIDS researchers, "a serious error in the interpretation of the epidemiological data. The CDC never wondered why 88% of the early Haitian AIDS cases in the United States occurred in males. In 1983 our

'Haitian children have been beaten up' group had identified risk factors, bisexuality and blood transfusion, in 79% of Haitian AIDS patients." [5]

Not until May 1985, nearly three years after its initial statement, did CDC officially withdraw its view [6]. Even then, Haitians still felt they were being officially victimised by the US authorities. "When the CDC removed Haitians from the list of risk groups, it refused to admit it had made an error", says Dr Pape. "Even now the CDC continues to stigmatise Haitians by preventing them from donating blood in the United States."

Haitian community workers in the United States reported that in some areas the unemployment rate for Haitians was twice that of other black workers, a situation they felt was directly attributable to AIDS. According to the AIDS Discrimination Unit of the New York City Commission on Human Rights in 1987: "Haitian children have been beaten up (and in at least one case, shot) in school; Haitian store owners have gone bankrupt as their businesses failed; and Haitian families have been evicted from their homes" [7].

Haitian tourism, before 1982 the country's second largest source of foreign earnings, fell from 70,000 visitors in the winter of 1981/2 to 10,000 the following year, according to Haitian government sources. At least six hotels had closed, with three more in financial trouble [8]. Haiti's tourism, which provided the second largest source of foreign income, has never recovered.

Battle of the blood tests

In 1983, at about the same time that the CDC put Haitians on the AIDS "risk group" list, Belgian and French physicians were seeing increasing numbers of immunodeficient central African patients who came to Europe in search of treatment for their unusual malady, soon to be identified as AIDS [9]. The doctors began to suspect that people might have been dying of AIDS in tropical Africa for many years, without attracting any special medical notice.

This was not an unreasonable speculation, as rare tropical diseases are sometimes carried back to developed countries. The musings of the medical profession were picked up and amplified in the press.

By the end of 1985, circumstantial evidence to support these beliefs seemed at hand. Results from the newly-developed blood test which could identify antibodies to the HIV virus were published by US researchers working on African blood samples. The samples were old ones, drawn from groups of patients in Kenya and Uganda in the 1960s and 1970s and stored for research purposes. When the US virologists tested these old samples for HIV antibodies, they found a very high percentage of positive results. Samples taken between 1980 and 1984 from the Turkana people of Kenya, for example, seemed to show that 59% were seropositive[10]. Blood samples drawn from Ugandan children in 1972-73 were taken as evidence that 66% were seropositive [11].

'*This was considered insulting by doctors in Africa*,'

These "false positive" results were thought to confirm that AIDS had existed for generations, and possibly centuries, in Central Africa. The researchers drew the false conclusion that infection with HIV had been widespread in Africa long before appearing in the United States or Europe. "I believe that the virus was present in Central Africa for a long period of time", Dr Robert Gallo, co-discoverer of the AIDS virus, told the *Los Angeles Times* in 1985 [12].

Gallo's statement was generally interpreted to mean that AIDS itself had long been present — unnoticed and undiagnosed by unobservant African physicians. This was considered insulting by doctors in Africa, and does not accord with the known facts. When cases of AIDS started appearing in African hospitals, local physicians quickly recognised that a new disease was responsible, and tried to identify it. The African doctors' resentment was increased by the way that some of the early blood samples had been collected: removed from African hospitals, and tested in the United States and Europe with little or no consultation with African researchers.

It has since become clear that the early testing technique was faulty [13] and better tests, employing different techniques, have since been developed [14]. These give far fewer "false-positive" results. There is now a strong current of opinion among scientists and others that the AIDS epidemic is as new to the African continent as it is to the rest of the world. A series of serological studies, using sensitive and specific blood tests, subject to experienced interpretation, has failed to find high prevalences of the AIDS virus in Africa before the mid-1970s, exactly the same situation as in the United States and Europe [15]. A single blood sample, drawn in Kinshasa, the capital of Zaire, in 1959, is the earliest known African sample to test positive for HIV using several different tests [16]. But as this is just one, very old sample, many researchers are disinclined to attach too much significance to it.

On the evidence available to date, the theory that AIDS as a disease was any more widespread in Africa than it was in the United States and Europe before the 1980s appears to be a premature conclusion reached on the basis of faulty bloodtests. But the political effects of this costly mistake stamped Central Africa as the birthplace of AIDS, leading to a still-smouldering epidemic of blame and counter-blame.

Where does AIDS come from?

When a new and deadly disease appears, it is natural to want to know where it comes from. But so far, we do *not* know the origins of HIV, the

'the medical profession started to track backwards' virus which causes AIDS. Much scientific effort (and far more non-scientific speculation) has been devoted to this question.

In theory it ought to be possible to find out when and where the first case of AIDS occurred. In practice, this is not so easy. The medical condition which was later to be called AIDS began to be noticed in the late 1970s and early 1980s in several widely separated locations, including Belgium, France, Haiti, the United States, Zaire, and Zambia.

As they learnt to diagnose AIDS, and in an effort to understand better just what they were up against, medical investigators in the United States and elsewhere began to look backwards in time, seeking the "first case" of the new disease. Step by step, this quest has led as far back as 1959, where the trail, for the present at least, runs cold.

The first medical reports of the syndrome soon to be named AIDS were published in the United States in June 1981 [17]. For two years preceding these reports, a small but growing number of physicians in New York City, Los Angeles and San Francisco were noticing in young homosexual men rare or unusual disease symptoms: pneumocystis pneumonia, Kaposi's sarcoma and a host of infections not found in otherwise healthy people. These ailments seemed to be related to an inexplicable deterioration in the men's immune systems [18].

Powerless to help these patients, or even to explain what had gone wrong with their bodies' defences, the doctors began to suspect the existence of a new, sexually transmitted infection.

Doctors at the US Centers for Disease Control in Atlanta, Georgia, started to wonder if blood transmission could also be a factor: similar symptoms were being recorded among intravenous drug users. By the end of 1981, records would later show that in the United States the disease had claimed the lives of 248 people.

Also in 1981, doctors in the Zairean capital of Kinshasa had begun to document dozens of cases where their patients' multiple infections seemed to relate to a collapse of the body's immune function [19]. And in Zambia the appearance of a new and more aggressive form of Kaposi's sarcoma, linked with immune deficiencies, prompted a physician working there to observe the similarity between the symptoms of her Zambian patients and those which had broken out among homosexuals in the United States [20]. As the medical profession started to track backwards through the 1970s, it became clear that some of the earliest known cases of AIDS had been seen by Belgian doctors in Africans. The first seems to have been a 34-year-old Zairean airline secretary, who flew to Belgium with her child late in 1977, to find out the reason for their persistent respiratory and intestinal infections [21].

Late 1980 and early 1981 saw doctors at a Parisian clinic baffled by cases of pneumocystis pneumonia in a Portuguese man recently arrived from Angola, in a Zairean woman, and in a French woman who had recently lived in Zaire [22]. Of the first 200 patients affected by the new disease in Europe, 42 were African [23].

In Haiti the tell-tale combination of Kaposi's sarcoma and uncontrollable opportunistic infections seems, in retrospect, to have first appeared in 1978-9 [24], coinciding with the earliest cases of Kaposi's sarcoma in homosexual men in the United States, and with the arrival in Europe of the first patients from Africa with the new disease. Haitian refugees with immunodeficiency disease were seen in increasing numbers in New York City and Miami during 1980/81. By mid-1982 the CDC had documented 34 such cases [25]. By October 1982 researchers in Haiti had diagnosed 61 cases.

The roughly simultaneous appearance of AIDS in the United States, Europe, Africa and Haiti prompted an obvious question: had AIDS been around for some time, unnoticed because the characteristic collection of opportunistic infections so indicative of underlying immune impairment had not been recognised?

After combing through medical histories of past patients, investigators found a small number of probable cases of AIDS going back nearly 30 years on three continents. Working back in time they found AIDS-like symptoms in patients as early as 1959:

- 1979: a 44-year-old homosexual man died with Kaposi's sarcoma in New York City [26].
- 1977: a 27-year-old Rwandan mother developed the novel immunodeficiency symptoms [27].
- 1977: the 34-year-old Zairean woman mentioned above who sought treatment in Belgium; she died in Kinshasa in 1978 [28].
- 1977: a 47-year-old Danish surgeon who had worked in rural Zaire died in Denmark [29].
- 1976: a 30-year-old Norwegian, his 33-year-old wife and their nine-year-old daughter all died after their health had deteriorated for seven to 10 years [30].
- 1975: a previously healthy seven-month-old black infant had pneumocystis in New York City [31].
- 1969: a 15-year-old black US boy died with Kaposi's sarcoma and opportunistic infections in St Louis, Missouri [32].
- 1959: a British sailor with Kaposi's sarcoma and pneumocystis died in Manchester, UK [33].
- 1959: a 45-year-old US man born in Haiti died [34].

In a few of these cases the retrospective diagnoses of AIDS are now supported by positive blood tests for HIV. Most, however, have been

'the early blood tests were discredited'
identified as possible early cases of AIDS on the basis of symptoms alone. The search goes on, and it is possible that even earlier possible cases will be found somewhere.

The further back in time such medical detective work extends, however, the more uncertain the retrospective diagnosis tends to become. People do not die of AIDS itself, for AIDS is not a disease but a syndrome: a mix of opportunistic infections which strike when immune functioning has been impaired by HIV. To determine retrospectively whether the infections that killed them were actually indications of AIDS is sometimes little more than guesswork.

African suspicions of the West

One of the first widely-publicised origins theories was that AIDS was an old African disease, and, as described above, the earliest examination of old blood samples led to the false conclusion that HIV had been endemic in Africa for decades. Physicians living and working in Africa found the suggestion that AIDS might have been present among their patients for years, unnoticed and undiagnosed, both improbable and insulting. When methods for testing blood for HIV antibodies improved, the early blood tests were discredited and it was accepted that AIDS was as new to Africa as it was to the United States and Europe.

One of the second most popular origins theories was that HIV had evolved from a parent virus, discovered in wild African green monkeys, passed to African people and thence to the rest of the world. Again, African scientists found the theory improbable, a view which seemed not unreasonable after the well-publicised evidence for the existence of an African green monkey virus turned out to be a case of mistaken identity on the part of US researchers (see "Tempest in a test tube" in Chapter Three).

Many Africans, and other people from the Third World, now regard with greatest scepticism any theories that AIDS originated in Africa. African journalists and commentators have found two general grounds for suspicion. The first is that the theories for the African origin of AIDS have often been accompanied by what they regard as ill-informed and racist speculation. The second is that much of the origins research seems to have been directed almost exclusively at Africa, and away from the major AIDS epidemics in the United States and Europe.

Another reason for the resentment felt by many African scientists towards Western AIDS research is the disparity between Africa and the West in access to the scientific and international media, and the difficulty African scientists have in getting international funding for their work.

Uganda, by illustration, one of the African countries both most affected by AIDS and most actively organising to combat it, was pledged

US$6.8 million by bilateral donors for the first year of its five-year AIDS programme, with international aid organisations promising US$20 million in June 1987 [35]. In comparison just one US university, Johns Hopkins in Baltimore, Maryland, had an AIDS research budget for 1987 alone of US$42 million, with an additional US$40 million for grants to other organisations and researchers.

'Africans saw the West as blaming AIDS on Africa.'

And while the United States, Europe and the Warsaw Pact countries spend US$500-600 per capita on health services, sub-Saharan Africa on average can afford only US$8. In Western Europe there is one doctor for every 470 patients; Zambia has one per 7,000 patients, and Uganda one per 21,000. While the United States has 123 medical schools and the United Kingdom has 31, Kenya, Uganda, Zaire and Zambia have only one each. The whole African continent has only 45 bio-medical journals, but 420 are published in the UK alone [36].

There is undoubtedly an enormous gap in scientific resources between developing African countries and the developed nations that have been setting the international AIDS research agenda.

This disparity, African scientists believe, makes it difficult for their views to reach an international audience. But the favourite target of African criticism has been the Western media.

Condemnation of Western reporting on AIDS has appeared widely in the African press, with articles which discuss promiscuity drawing particularly acid responses. It was a "campaign of systematic denigration against black Africa" said the Cameroon newspaper *La Gazette* in July 1987 [37]; it "deliberately encourages racism and reinforces racist ideologies", said the Ivory Coast newspaper, *Fraternité-Matin* in August 1987 [38]. *New Vision* in Uganda referred to "Western escapism and racist hangups" [39].

The idea that AIDS had started in Africa was repeatedly denounced: it was reminiscent of a "colonial mentality which capitalises on our weakness and underdevelopment to attribute everything that is bad and negative to the so-called dark continent", said Lt-Col Abdul Mumini Aminu, governor of the Nigerian state of Borno, in 1987 [40].

Just as Africans saw the West as blaming AIDS on Africa, some of them now blamed it back on the West. "Today pornography in Western cities conveys a lurid tale of a society which has gone berserk in its sexual habits [with] negative consequences for world public health", wrote a correspondent in the Nigerian magazine *African Concord* in January 1987. Westerners had brought AIDS to Africa with their "weird sexual propositions" [41] — a view echoed by *La Gazette* in July 1987, which referred to Westerners coming to Africa with their "sexual perversions" [42]. "Many of the venereal diseases now found in Kenya", said an editorial in the Kenyan *Standard*, "were brought into the country by the same foreigners who are now waging a smear campaign against us" [43].

Blame hinders AIDS campaigns

"African AIDS 'deadly threat to Britain'" ran the headline of the front-page story of the British *Sunday Telegraph* on 21 September 1986, in a classic instance of Europeans blaming Africa for AIDS. The article claimed that an investigation into the potential risks to Britain posed by AIDS in Africa, ordered by the British foreign secretary, had resulted in "a series of alarming reports" from British high commissions in Tanzania, Uganda and Zambia. British diplomats, the story said, warned that African visitors to Britain "could be a primary source of infection and should be subject to compulsory tests".

"It would be monstrous," the *Sunday Telegraph* said, "if ministers were to hold back from action lest they be accused of racial discrimination. For in this instance there is a positive duty to discriminate. In the matter of AIDS", it asserted, "Black Africa does have

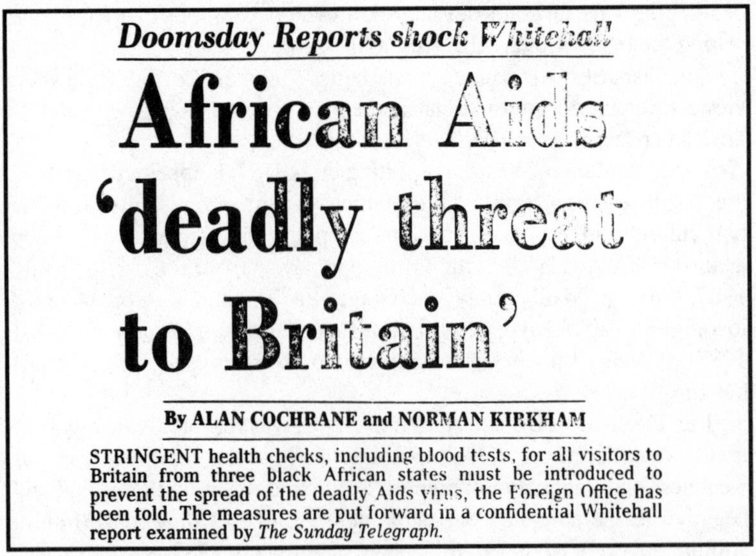

Figure 6.2
This British newspaper headline (*Sunday Telegraph* 21 September 1986) was followed by a story calling for blood tests for all visitors, especially students, from three African countries. Such press coverage was seen in Africa as racist, and seriously held back essential international co-operation against the AIDS epidemic.

Doomsday Reports shock Whitehall

African Aids 'deadly threat to Britain'

By ALAN COCHRANE and NORMAN KIRKHAM

STRINGENT health checks, including blood tests, for all visitors to Britain from three black African states must be introduced to prevent the spread of the deadly Aids virus, the Foreign Office has been told. The measures are put forward in a confidential Whitehall report examined by *The Sunday Telegraph*.

a uniquely bad record" [44]. Within a few weeks, the United Kingdom let it be known that there were no plans to screen Zambians, after strong behind-the-scenes pressure from the UK health department and its medical advisers. From a public health point of view, to test a few score black Zambians a year, and not to test the hundreds of thousands of white US tourists who visit Britain annually, was seen by many British AIDS workers as absurd and racist.

But the damage had been done. Zambia's minister of health reacted quickly to the suggestion that Zambians, notably students, should be screened for the AIDS virus on entering Britain: "We will study the situation, and we may reciprocate in the same way if Britain goes ahead.

After all, AIDS is a capitalist disease which is not only common in Zambia but throughout the world." [45]

The screening apparently contemplated by the British Government was seen as a political insult in Zambia, where a number of British physicians and researchers had been working in collaboration with Zambian colleagues on AIDS-related projects.

An immediate consequence was some delay in plans to screen Zambian blood supplies: while health officials were determined to do this, political support for action on AIDS was still limited, and the UK testing row undermined it.

'there was an unwritten rule not to discuss AIDS in Zambia'

Zambian officials worried about the consequences on tourism of the *Sunday Telegraph* story, particularly since the majority of tourists were European. The year 1986 had been an all-time low for the Zambian tourist trade, with revenues down nearly 25% from 1985. Officials believed that an important factor was "negative publicity campaigns in our traditional tourist markets" [46].

Following the *Sunday Telegraph* story, British researchers received a letter from a Zambian official which read in part: "I regret to inform you that the mass media in recent weeks have raised problems which require questions to be asked as to whether collaboration should be continued with outside researchers. I am afraid that we are in a political world, and such matters, as they are reported in the British press, make it difficult to continue." [47]

Zambia is not the only country to reconsider joint AIDS endeavours due to media coverage judged to be unfavourable. The first international conference on AIDS, held in Brussels in 1985, was boycotted by some African states which anticipated that research on the green monkey hypothesis would be presented. Scientists working on Zaire's AIDS research programme, for instance, were refused government permission to present the results of their work at the conference. Many African researchers who had booked to go to the conference pulled out at the last minute, and of those who did go, several held a press briefing to contest strenuously that the evidence pointed to an African origin for the AIDS virus.

The international climate of accusation and blame which has shadowed more constructive approaches to the AIDS pandemic has put a number of governments on the defensive. In some cases they have refused to talk about AIDS abroad, and discouraged talk about AIDS at home. Newspapers in some African countries now openly acknowledge that AIDS was until recently something to keep quiet about. "A few years ago," said the *Times of Zambia* in August 1987, "there was an unwritten rule not to discuss the presence of AIDS in Zambia so as not to discourage tourists from coming here. It was a policy of the ministry of health not to alarm the public." [48]

The same applied to Nigeria, according to the Nigerian magazine *Newswatch* in March 1987. "In the six years since the AIDS scourge spread across the world, Nigeria has tried its best to wish it away. No co-ordinated efforts were made to find out whether or not the disease was already present in Nigeria, and if so, how to contain it. Not until last year did [the health minister] first send a five-man team to Geneva to learn the basics of coping with the disease ... the federal government is now scrambling to cover lost ground." [49]

Exasperated at what they saw as exaggeration of their AIDS statistics, or wanting to play down the degree of infection, some African governments banned AIDS researchers and physicians from talking to the press. "One result of such attempts at control," said James Brooke, West African correspondent for the *New York Times*, in November 1987, "has been to force foreign reporters to rely more heavily on foreign researchers working in those countries, making it more difficult than before to convey an authentically African point of view" [50].

As the above examples show, blame and counter-blame are not only unpleasant; they contribute to delays in vital preventive programmes and, therefore, in saving lives. President Kenneth Kaunda of Zambia, announcing in October 1987 that his son Masuzyo had died of AIDS, said it best: "What is more important than knowing where this disease came from is knowing where it is going... There is nothing to hide."

Many of the issues covered in Chapter Six are dealt with in more detail in Blaming Others: Prejudice, race and worldwide AIDS, *by Renée Sabatier et al (Panos, London & Washington DC, 1988).*

CHAPTER SEVEN

AIDS AND THE DEVELOPMENT DOLLAR

The AIDS epidemic is not just an economic burden. It mainly affects, in terms of social and economic development, the most vital segment of the population: adults between 20 and 49 years old. In Third World communities the loss of these young adults can be disproportionately damaging.

Fewer Third World teenagers have opportunities for higher education than those in developed countries, and when educated people in the 20-49 age group die, they are much less easily replaced. Dr Jonathan Mann, head of WHO's global programme on AIDS, warns of the "potential for economic and political destabilisation in areas of the developing world most affected by HIV. What political system could withstand the ultimate destabilising impact of a 20% or 25% or higher infection rate among young adults?"[1]

In urban areas in some sub-Saharan countries, up to 25% of young adults are *already* HIV carriers, with rates among those reporting to clinics for sexually transmitted diseases passing 30%, and among female prostitutes up to 90% [2].

Among adults in Kinshasa, Zaire, there are 55-100 new cases of AIDS per 100,000 population every year [3]. By comparison, in New York City, the annual incidence in adults in 1986 was 110 per 100,000 for men and 12 per 100,000 for women [4].

New York City's epidemic is thus roughly comparable in size with that of Kinshasa, but New York's financial and medical resources are many times greater. The whole of Zaire depends on one large teaching hospital in Kinshasa as a centre for both treatment and medical expertise, while New York has dozens of comparable facilities. And whereas Kinshasa is the political, economic, commercial, military and transport heart of Zaire, New York is but one of many equivalent centres in the United States. New York also benefits from US federal government funding for AIDS research and treatment, which is targeted to exceed US$1 billion for 1989, a sum three times greater than the total annual foreign assistance from all sources received by Zaire in 1987.

In some central African hospitals a quarter to a third of scarce hospital beds are occupied by AIDS patients [5], while even in less heavily-affected Costa Rica officials have predicted that a similar percentage of beds could be taken by AIDS patients by the mid-1990s [6].

Figure 7.1
A priest in rural Uganda visits a 45-year-old man dying from AIDS; his 30-year-old wife also has the disease. The impact of AIDS on social and economic development in the Third World may be critical, because unlike most other diseases it hits not the very young and the old, but men and women in their most productive years.

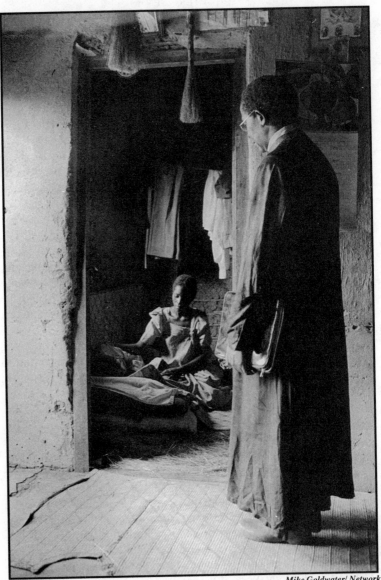

Mike Goldwater/ Network

Reversing health gains

In cities of several central African countries, 5-25% of women in their child-bearing years have been found to be seropositive [7]. The transmission of HIV from infected mothers to their infants means that, as in New York and some other US cities, some African cities are now in the early stages of a new wave of AIDS, this time in young children.

The growing proportion of AIDS cases attributed to heterosexual transmission in a number of Caribbean countries points in the same direction. No one yet knows the extent to which heterosexual transmission elsewhere will cause cases of infant AIDS.

'Child AIDS threatens Africa's position'

For much of this century, one of the most important indicators of a country's progress in health matters has been the rate at which infant mortality has been reduced. In developed countries, the dangers of disease and malnutrition during the first years of life have been transformed. Today, deaths of children under five in these countries constitute only 3% of total deaths. Progress in the richest countries has been so remarkable that a low child mortality rate has become a "gold standard" of development: one of the measures thought to best portray a country's overall social and economic progress.

For the world as a whole, infant mortality rates declined by 51% from the 1950s to the 1980s [8], a trend projected to continue to the end of the century, with progress among developing countries most evident in South-East Asia. Nevertheless, between 1980 and 1985, 98% of deaths in children under five were in the Third World. The statistics are starkest in Africa, where 40% of all deaths still occur among young children. Moreover, Africa's share of total world infant deaths is expected to increase over the next decade. While progress in reducing infant mortality has been made in a number of African countries, the continent's position relative to other parts of the developing world is worsening, and the absolute number of children dying is increasing.

Child AIDS threatens to erode Africa's position still further, and may "tragically cancel the achievements of past decades"[9] in maternal and child health programmes. Infant mortality is on the rise even in some of the world's richest countries. The United States, with much of its large population of minority racial and ethnic groups living in "Third World" conditions, currently ranks behind 18 other countries in infant mortality, including Singapore and] Spain. Children of its black and Latino minorities are worse off than those in Bulgaria, Costa Rica or Cuba [10]. Child AIDS is growing so rapidly among these US groups that it may soon become the largest single cause of infant death nationwide. Heterosexually transmitted AIDS already affects, or may soon affect, progress in child health in other parts of the world.

It has often been suggested that, since AIDS predominantly affects young adults, dependency ratios — the balance between economically productive adults and the dependent young and old — would rise in hard-hit regions. AIDS may cause mortality rates among the economically and socially most productive age groups to double, triple or rise even higher [11], meaning that each surviving adult would have to support a larger number of children and elderly dependents, and making economic growth less likely.

*'to
question
the ability
of the
existing
health
system'*

But recent research based on a computer model of AIDS epidemiology in some developing countries has contradicted this early prediction. Mortality from AIDS among adults in heavily affected regions is likely to be fierce, the study shows, but dependency ratios will remain unchanged because the number of deaths among young children with AIDS will be much greater than has yet been realised [12].

The cost of treatment

By 1991 one out of every four hospital beds in New York City will be occupied by an AIDS patient [13], a proportion already approached in major hospitals in some cities in Central Africa [14]. How much will it cost to treat these patients? In the United States and some other developed countries the direct lifetime costs of treating each PWA (person with AIDS) have been calculated, giving figures so high as to call into question the ability of the existing health system to sustain them. Caring for each US PWA will cost around US$65,000 from diagnosis to death, and the direct costs of caring for the total predicted number of AIDS cases will reach an annual US$8.56 billion by 1991. By that time 5.9 million hospital bed-days will be occupied by PWAs: twice the number occupied by lung cancer patients, the second leading cause of death nationwide [15].

It is obvious that in cash terms the amount spent on treating PWAs in Third World countries cannot possibly reach the sums spent in industrialised countries. Brazilian spending per patient is estimated to average US$21,500 [16]; that in Mexico US$7,345 [17]; in Zaire US$816 [18]; and in Tanzania US$367 [19].

These sums roughly parallel the size of each country's GNP: the amount spent treating AIDS patients in each country is thus directly related to the quantity of available resources.

AIDS is an expensive illness, and the true extent of its impact depends on the resources a nation can make available for treatment, prevention, education and research. Even taking into account its large number of AIDS cases, the United States is in a strong economic position to combat its AIDS epidemic.

In many AIDS-affected countries in Africa, annual per capita health spending is less than the cost of a single HIV blood test. The disproportion between per capita AIDS cases and per capita income (gross national product per person) in developing countries is shown in Figure 7.2. Column one shows each country's AIDS epidemic as a percentage of the US epidemic, measured in cases per million population. Column two shows national per capita income, again expressed as a percentage of US per capita income.

Column three shows an AIDS Resources Index: column two as a

Figure 7.2

AIDS RESOURCES INDEX

Country	AIDS epidemic	Per capita income %	AIDS resources index %
Sweden	9	71	809
Switzerland	25	98	392
France	25	57	233
Mexico	6	12	209
Brazil	8	10	125
USA	**100**	**100**	**100**
Zimbabwe	5	4	86
Trinidad	66	36	55
Honduras	12	4	36
Zaire	4	1	26
Dominican Rep.	29	5	16
Kenya	25	2	7
Zambia	40	2	6
Rwanda	0	2	3
Uganda	56	1	2
Haiti	83	2	2

Column one shows cases of AIDS per million population as a percentage of the US total per million [51]. Column two shows GNP per capita as a percentage of the US GNP per capita [52]. Column three is column two divided by column one, expressed as a percentage.

percentage of column one. This is a crude estimation of the resources a country can make available for combating its AIDS epidemic.

With all its limitations, the table makes some interesting points. Sweden and Switzerland and France have two to eight times more economic resources available per case of AIDS than does the United States, and Mexico has twice more.

At the bottom end of the table, Zambia, Rwanda, Uganda and Haiti are already finding AIDS 15-50 times more of an economic burden than the United States.

Does this mean that a PWA in New York or California receives better treatment than an AIDS patient in Trinidad or Zambia? This is a question which has yet to be answered precisely. Clearly, the cash cost of treatment in hospitals in the United States is inflated by, for example,

Sister Nellie in Kampala

The city of Kampala is swelling as citizens who fled the capital during the past bloody years return. With the returnees comes HIV, the virus that causes AIDS, locally dubbed 'slim disease'. Everyone in Kampala knows about 'slim'; most people have seen relatives or friends die of it.

Sister Nelezinha Carvalho is a Ugandan nun who trained as a medical technician in Britain. She heads the laboratory at St Francis General and Maternity Hospital, working with a team of 11 Ugandan lab technicians and a dozen students each year. They have trained with her despite shortages of classrooms, textbooks, equipment and even electricity to provide light for reading. Sister Nellie is part of Uganda's national AIDS committee.

The first edition of this dossier in November 1986 described how Sister Nellie and medical colleagues began to notice that some of their patients had AIDS in late 1985. Concerned about the potential contamination of transfusion blood supplies by the AIDS virus, Sister Nellie flew to Britain to learn how to perform the lab test which allows screening of donated blood. Returning to Kampala in May 1986, she brought with her a dozen bulky boxes: the equipment necessary to perform the tests, including a US$3,000 electronic blood analysis machine. But Uganda's supplies were so depleted after the war that she also had to bring back sundry items such as rubber gloves, lab coats, test tubes, bottles and plastic tubing.

Sister Nellie and her assistant, William Wamale, immediately began testing the hospital's stored blood, but shortages of basic supplies were so common that they had to work bare-handed. They took the risk of contracting the virus should they accidentally cut themselves on a piece of glass. Even disinfecting the lab was difficult, since everyday household bleach, which kills the virus quickly, was often unavailable. Now there is bleach, but due to long-term repairs on Kampala's water system, water is in short supply, and plans to use a WHO-supplied steriliser have had to be postponed.

Today one in five of the samples tested is found to be positive for antibodies to HIV. An average of 50 requests per day come in from doctors needing blood tests to make a diagnosis. People going abroad also come to be tested, and the lab screens blood for hospitals within a 60 mile (96 kilometre) radius. The lab team estimate that since 1986 they have tested over 10,000 blood samples for HIV. Facilities at St Francis are splitting at the seams. The small lab, housing Sister Nellie and close to 30 team members, is adjacent to the always-crowded waiting room of the outpatient clinic. The hospital has agreed to build a new, high-standard lab with facilities for a blood bank and screening, staff training, research and data processing. The estimated cost is US$349,000, but Sister Nellie is hoping that a total of US$4 million can eventually be raised to support the hospital and its work.

Since her story first appeared in the Panos dossier, Sister Nellie reports that people from a number of developed countries have "been so very generous and sent us supplies and even monthly donations stemming from special fund raising drives". This response has enabled St Francis to set up a mobile home care unit for AIDS patients who have been discharged from hospital. "Conditions are improving", Sister Nellie says, "but there is still so much to do. The new lab is just a dream, but we hope and trust that it will soon become a reality."

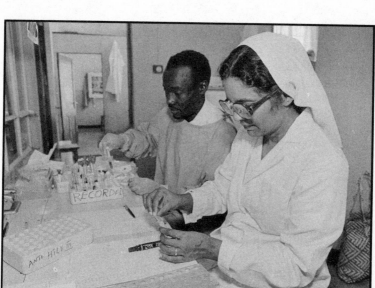

Figure 7.3
Sister Nellie
Carvalho and her
assistant William
Wamale do HIV
tests at St Francis
General and
Maternity Hospital,
Kampala, Uganda.
They have often
lacked protective
laboratory supplies
like bleach and
rubber gloves while
they handle infected
blood.

Mike Goldwater/ Network

higher medical salaries, higher malpractice insurance and higher capital equipment costs than apply in the Third World.

However, in general terms it is clear that certain life-prolonging treatments, such as the drug AZT, cost too much to be used in the Third World. Shortages of less novel medicines such as antibiotics are also routinely experienced in lower income nations. And shortages of syringes, disinfectants, rubber gloves, running water, electricity and other items hamper treatment in Third World hospitals.

AIDS and the economy

The indirect costs of AIDS in Third World countries cannot yet be forecast accurately, but the impact of the epidemic on social and economic development may be critical. How will premature deaths due to the disease affect national productivity and income? How will key sectors of the economy in different countries fare? Prediction is difficult due to lack of basic data, but a preliminary study by researchers at Harvard University suggested that economic losses due to AIDS in five seriously-affected central African countries might begin to exceed total foreign aid to those countries by 1991 [20].

In some countries key industries may be jeopardised. Zambia's Copperbelt, a region that produces 20% of Zambia's gross national product with just 6% of its labour force, faces labour losses due to AIDS, which Zambian researchers believe could damage the viability of the

'*AIDS robs countries of their young adults*' whole industry [21]. Nearly half of those employed in mining are men between 20 and 44 years of age, typically married and with several children. Zambian researchers point out that AIDS must be regarded as a "family disease", as likely to affect wives and infants as the young men employed in mining and other industries. Since the mining industry pays not only for the education and training of the miners, but for all-encompassing health and social services for their families, the financial impact of AIDS on this key sector of Zambia's economy may soon threaten its viability [22].

Such national economic losses are accompanied by hardship on a human scale. In a number of African cultures mourning takes the form of lengthy funeral ceremonies which numerous family members gather to attend. A Zairean family, one of whose children has died of AIDS, may spend up to the equivalent of a year's income on the funeral and interment [23]. And increasingly in those parts of Africa where AIDS has become widely-recognised and feared, families are spending household income on traditional cures, quack remedies and faith healers in a desperate search for treatments for those suffering the disease.

Lost productivity

AIDS robs affected countries of their young adults: can this theft be quantified in economic terms, relative to losses from other common diseases? A group of African and Western researchers have calculated that, in terms of years of economically productive life lost, AIDS already ranks fifth of 13 diseases common in several African countries, ahead of malaria, measles, pneumonia and tuberculosis [24]. For each case of HIV infection which occurs, an average of 8.8 years of productive healthy life is lost, more than for all but four other diseases: sickle cell anaemia, malnutrition, birth injuries and infant tetanus. The indirect economic impact of AIDS is thus heavy, ranking intermediate between childhood and adult diseases (because AIDS strikes both adults and children in Africa).

In the United States, economists have estimated that the cost to industry of illness and death due to AIDS will have totalled US$55,000 million by 1991 [25]. Lifetime loss of earned income for each individual struck by AIDS in the United States is estimated at US$207,639, the equivalent of 12.4 times GNP per capita. In Zaire the comparable figure is US$1,780 per person with AIDS (10.4 times GNP per capita), and in Tanzania US$3,759 (13.0 times GNP per capita) [26].

Such an impact could not come at a worse time. Both national and per capita incomes in many African countries have been falling for several years, with the economies of some countries, for example Zambia, contracting by nearly half. As a continent, Africa is staggering under a foreign debt load described by UN Secretary-General Javier Perez de Cuellar as "the most serious balance of payment crisis in the history of the region" [27].

'fears have led govern- ments to suppress their AIDS figures'

AIDS and tourism

Tourism figures prominently in the economic plans of Third World governments. It is one of the major means by which many hope to stem the global flow of cash from South to North — in 1987 US$30 billion more flowed in that direction than the other way around. With the world's population ever more mobile, attracting a bigger share of the cash-rich, footloose travellers who journey to foreign parts each year is seen as an unmissable opportunity to grab precious foreign exchange.

Tourism in the age of AIDS has become a controversial business. Governments with great expectations for the growth of their tourist industries have been infuriated by press reports which point to AIDS in their countries. After a headline suggesting that Zambian students who might be infected with HIV posed a "deadly threat to Britain" appeared in the British press in 1986 [28], Zambian officials worried that their tourist trade might suffer, especially since the majority of the tourists were European. The year 1986 was an all-time low for the trade, with revenues down nearly 25% from 1985. Although political instability in the southern African region and international currency fluctuations contributed to this decline, Zambian officials believed that an important factor was "negative publicity campaigns in our traditional tourist markets" [29].

The Kenyan Government has also been nervous about AIDS stories. In November 1985 it had banned an issue of the *International Herald Tribune* that discussed high levels of HIV infection found among Nairobi prostitutes [30]. The prostitutes' HIV status was a continuing source of irritation for at least a year, during which time government spokesmen denied the medical findings and accused those reporting them of bias [31]. Some of the reports were said to have led to a large drop in hotel bookings by German tourists.

The same fears have led many governments to suppress or adjust their AIDS figures. The example of Haiti seemed to provide grounds for anxiety. Shortly after researchers in the United States linked Haitians with AIDS, US visitors dropped from 70,000 to 10,000 within a year [32]. Before the epidemic tourism was the country's second largest source of income in a precarious economy, directly and indirectly supporting 25,000 jobs [33].

Yet tourists are generally at no greater risk from AIDS abroad than they are in their own countries. As the president of the Canadian aid agency, CIDA, graphically put it in early 1987: AIDS "does not jump

'boys are paid for sex with foreign tourists'

out of trees at visiting tourists or businessmen" [34]. It is transmitted in exactly the same ways in the Third World as anywhere else.

Sex tourism

For both visitors and the host country, tourism becomes a risky business when tours and sex are sold together. In some cases, as in Thailand, a country's tourist industry is heavily based on the packaged sex holiday, catering for those who go abroad to do things they would probably never do at home. But in most cases the sale of sexual services is less obvious, the result of the drawing power of the dollar and other hard currencies in tourist hotels, bars and other haunts. For some young, under-educated and unemployed local inhabitants, prostitution in exchange for dollars or favours may be the only available means of survival, and, they hope, a means of advancement. In the Philippines young women entertain US servicemen; in Sri Lanka boys are paid for sex with foreign tourists; in the United States men and women sell their bodies to pay for drugs; in Brazil and Italy *travestis* (transvestites) seek cash for sex in order to earn the money for sex-change operations; in Kenya young women may exchange sex for money or favours as they look for a husband; in Thailand teenagers support their families by dancing in go-go bars.

Developments in Tanzania are typical of those taking place in many parts of Africa, in the years of recession and sluggish economic growth since the 1973 OPEC oil embargo. Increased sexual activity with multiple partners, especially with strangers and foreigners who can afford to pay more, has become a means of survival for growing numbers of young women in urban areas. Research by the University of Dar es Salaam has shown that prostitution in the capital has been increasing at about 20% a year since the early 1980s. According to this research, 70% of those who work in the sex trade are dependent for their economic survival on the income they earn from prostitution [35].

Haiti provides a chilling example of the spread of AIDS through tourism. Haitian researchers have accumulated evidence, through analysis of Haitian blood samples going back over a decade, which they believe shows that the AIDS virus arrived in Haiti with North American tourists. While large numbers of tourists visited briefly from cruise ships, the majority of those who stayed in Haiti were homosexual men, who paid for sex with local men who had wives or girlfriends and considered themselves heterosexual. First the bisexual men became infected, then their female partners, and now Haiti has a full-scale heterosexual AIDS epidemic on its hands.

The neighbouring country of the Dominican Republic, another favoured holiday destination for homosexual men from the United States, has seen a similar shift from homosexual to heterosexual transmission.

The Costa Rican authorities have begun to screen foreign students and applicants for residence for HIV antibodies, because they fear that Costa Rica could follow the Haitian and Dominican model.

Thailand has one of the world's most open and thriving sex industries. Its major cities and holiday resorts depend heavily on tourism, which brings in over US$1 billion dollars a year [36]. In order to attract visitors, it spent US$170 million in 1987 [37]. In the same year blood survey results of more than 15,000 sex workers showed that 2.6% of male prostitutes and 0.03% of female prostitutes tested positive for HIV [38].

In the Philippines five of every six people known to be infected is a hospitality worker connected to the US military bases. Although the US Government now guarantees that all servicemen abroad have tested seronegative, there is no screening of the thousands of tourists who fly to Manila, where young boys and girls are easily available. In 1985 the Philippines earned US$507 million from tourism [39].

In Indonesia companions to tourists who have fallen ill have themselves contracted the virus [40]. Indonesia's tourist revenue almost doubled between 1981 and 1985, representing almost US$500 million in annual earnings [41]. Sri Lankan health ministry officials have estimated that 10% of tourists arriving in the country have sexual contacts with locals [42]. As tourists travel further afield, such countries as the small island nations of the Pacific join those of the Caribbean in seeing themselves at great risk.

Larger countries also fear the spread of the AIDS virus through travel. At Carnival time in Brazil, leaflets in four languages have been handed

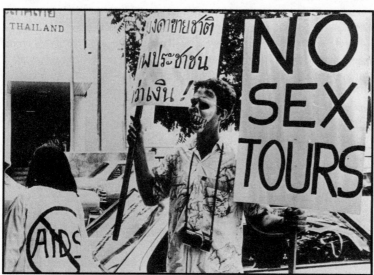

Edgar Mac Tressin/ Gamma

Figure: 7.4 Protesters determined to stop "sex tours" to Thailand demonstrate against the tourist authority in Bangkok. They argue that the Thai government spends too little on AIDS prevention and too much on attracting unattached men on packaged holidays in which sex is a major attraction. Foreign tourism earns Thailand over US$ 1,000 million a year.

Figure: 7.5 US sailors jubilantly pour off the carrier Midway after docking in the Philippines for R & R (rest and relaxation). The belief that military personnel have infected nearly 50 local "hospitality girls" has led Philippine authorities to demand that all foreign seamen present "AIDS clearance certificates" approved by the government.

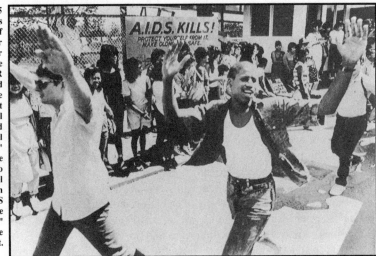

Willie Salenga/ NYT Pictures

to incoming tourists at airports, urging them to use condoms. A theme of Sweden's national AIDS awareness campaign has been to encourage Swedes to think about their sexual behaviour when they travel: "Remember that *AIDS is spreading*, both in Sweden and abroad." A similar theme has been struck in the British slogan: "When you go away, AIDS doesn't."

The responsibility for transmitting AIDS lies less with prostitutes than with their clients. Women who offer sexual services in cities as different as Glasgow [43] and Nairobi [44] have shown themselves willing to adopt condoms if approached by the right education campaign. However, even where condoms are easily available and prostitutes want to use them, a client who is older, offers more money or is physically more powerful may insist on unprotected sex [45].

For Third World governments whose citizens have increasing material expectations, as for those less well off who are walking an economic tightrope, the choice between tourism and the risk of AIDS is a pernicious one. Long-term, the solution may be to escape from dependence on the type of tourism in which sexual services play a predominant role. Some Third World commentators have argued against dependence on tourism, which they believe is merely false development anyway; it "is a fantasy because it does not create real wealth. It brings money quickly only to a few people." [46]

Given a choice, many of those who live in Third World countries would prefer other routes to development. In a recent public opinion survey conducted in the Tanzanian capital of Dar es Salaam, 20% of those interviewed believed that AIDS should be controlled by banning prostitution, and by offering the prostitutes alternative employment through the institution of small-scale programmes and government training schemes [47].

More and more, the young women and men whose livelihoods depend on some form of prostitution are reacting against the exploitation in which they find themselves, demanding that governments find ways to create jobs which they can perform with safety and dignity. Thai women demonstrating in Bangkok have demanded that money spent on attracting tourists from overseas should be directed towards rural poverty and AIDS prevention [48]. They say that the Thai Government spends 20 times as much each year on tourism promotion as it does on its AIDS prevention activities [49].

'the government spends 20 times as much on tourism as it does on AIDS'

The roots of the present Thai sex industry can be traced back to the regular influx of dollar-rich US soldiers on leave from the Vietnam war. Western influence elsewhere in the Third World, first through colonialism and now through tourism, is perceived by many in developing countries to have been similarly undermining. Ugandan President, Yoweri Museveni, who has taken a strong personal lead in AIDS education in his country, has stated that the impact of Europe on Africa has had damaging effects on traditional African sexual morality. AIDS "is the result of European influences — European liberalism, which is good in some respects, has brought a lot of permissiveness, which in a backward society is dangerous" [50].

CHAPTER EIGHT

THE INTERNATIONAL STRATEGY

"Tell us what needs to be done — not the way things are usually done. It is not "business as usual" at the Global Programme on AIDS, and has not been since the programme was founded"
— Dr Jonathan Mann, director, WHO global programme on AIDS, February 1988.

W HO held its first meeting on AIDS at its Geneva headquarters in late 1983. In the three years of preliminary activity between that meeting and the setting up of WHO's special AIDS programme in February 1987, it became apparent that, if AIDS were to be stopped, a global effort was required. AIDS was first diagnosed in 1981. Given the crisis it has come to represent, why was this realisation so long in coming?

Within WHO, as within every body that has been confronted with AIDS since the pandemic began, individual and institutional attitudes were a crucial factor. AIDS is in many ways a unique health challenge: the infection is invisible, insidious, and takes a long time to produce disease. It is transmitted sexually, a fact which makes it difficult to discuss freely. And it is new, requiring those who have been intensely committed to improving health in other areas to accept that their programmes might be radically affected by the demands arising from AIDS control efforts. So within WHO itself, and within the bureaucracies of its member governments, coming to grips with the idea and the reality of AIDS took time.

Very early on, WHO staff recall, there was a small group of countries which voiced concern to WHO and urged action. But a greater number of member states were less keen and so WHO, following the majority, adopted an incremental approach, moving slowly from meeting to meeting and stage to stage. The turning point came in late 1986, with the establishment of what was then known as WHO's special programme on AIDS (see Figure 8.1).

From this point on, the climate of world opinion on AIDS seemed to change almost overnight, like a liquid in which a seed crystal has been planted. Not every country with an AIDS epidemic would publicly acknowledge that this was the case; throughout 1987 some countries continued to have mixed reactions, with denial still gaining the upper hand. But the tide had turned, and it was clear that those countries were finding themselves part of a rapidly shrinking minority.

It is undeniable that WHO itself was slow to mobilise on AIDS, as WHO director-general Dr Halfdan Mahler has admitted. He has identified denial as one of the chief causes of delay in the international response to the AIDS pandemic and said pointedly and courageously: "I know that many people at first refused to believe that a crisis was upon us. I know because I was one of them [1]".

In addition to the evolution of attitudes over the period 1983-7, WHO had to grapple with the sheer scale of the effort that would be needed to bring the AIDS pandemic under control. Worldwide programmes to control or eliminate specific diseases were themselves a relatively new concept, implemented for the first time with the global campaign to eradicate smallpox, begun in earnest in 1967 and declared successful in 1980.

The war on smallpox cost US$81 million [2]. In November 1986, WHO's global AIDS co-ordinating office consisted of one physician, one secretary and an official budget of only US$580,000 a year. Today full-time and part-time AIDS staff in Geneva number almost 100, with a global programme budget of US$22 million (1987) rising to US$66 million (1988). This means that funding for WHO's Global Programme on AIDS (GPA) will have exceeded, in the programme's first two years of existence, WHO's entire 14-year budget for smallpox eradication.

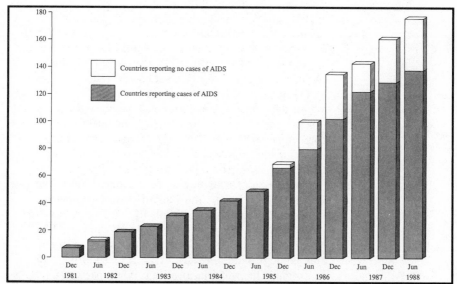

Figure 8.1: As AIDS has spread, more and more countries have started to report cases to WHO. Those countries shown as reporting no cases have established an AIDS surveillance system. Source: WHO

'1987 was the year of global AIDS mobilisation'

WHO's commitment, and that of its member states, to global AIDS control is substantial. Projections are that it will have to grow in financial terms to US$650 million by 1991.

In just 18 months of unprecedented activity, Dr Jonathan Mann, the programme's director, and his staff have firmly established WHO as the directing and co-ordinating agency of the global offensive against AIDS. Mann calls 1987, the year when the GPA was formally launched, "the year of global AIDS mobilisation" [3]. At the centre of a whirlwind of country visits, consultations, meetings, briefings, conferences, speeches, interviews and articles, he and the programme staff have made an impact which is becoming evident in virtually every corner of the globe. This was the picture by mid-1988:

● 176 countries have joined WHO's global AIDS reporting network — nearly 40 of them reporting *before* any national AIDS cases had occured.

● 151 countries have established national AIDS committees, with national AIDS programmes now in place in nearly all the nations of sub-Saharan Africa, and in more than 30 Asian, Caribbean and Latin American countries.

● The global strategy against AIDS put forward by WHO has received the endorsement of, among others, the World Health Assembly, the UN General Assembly, the UN Economic and Social Council and the 1987 Venice summit of Western political leaders.

● WHO has convened more than 30 consultations of international experts on important AIDS issues, been producing policy statements on a range of sensitive and sometimes controversial topics, such as whether countries should screen visitors for HIV antibodies. (See Box later in this chapter: "WHO Consensus Statements")

● Within the UN family, WHO is collaborating with several other agencies to improve their joint efficiency in combating AIDS: with UNICEF (harmonising policies on childhood immunisation and breastfeeding); with the United Nations Development Programme (co-ordination of activities at the national level in the Third World); with the United Nations Fund for Population Activities (on the role of family planners in AIDS prevention); with UNESCO (developing AIDS education for schools); with the World Bank (economic and demographic impact); with ILO (politics and education in the workplace); with FAO (impact on food production); and with the World Tourism Organisation (information for travellers).

Pulse points in a global network

National AIDS committees are the pulse points of a rapidly-developing global AIDS surveillance and control network. By July 1988 more than 170 countries had asked WHO to collaborate in their national programmes, and GPA staff had criss-crossed the globe on over 300 consultative missions to assist them. One hundred and two countries now have short-term (6-12 month) national AIDS plans; 30 medium-term (3-5 year) plans are complete. Most of the medium-term plans have been devised with developing countries.

'in many Third World countries annual capita healtrh budgets are less than the cost of a hamburger'

What is involved in drawing up such a plan? The process sounds straightforward until it is remembered that in vast parts of the world a health care system — a functional framework of trained health workers and educators, operative clinics, laboratories and hospitals which is accessible to the entire population at an affordable cost — is virtually non-existent. Haiti and Uganda, for example, have both been hit hard by AIDS. Both have experienced years of political turmoil which have all but destroyed their transport, communications, administrative and health infrastructures. "To be successful in countries such as these we are literally going to have to revive the entire health system", says Dr Daniel Tarantola, who heads the GPA unit which supports national AIDS activities [4].

Tarantola describes the practical difficulties he and those working within the countries encountered daily: "There might be a health unit with one or several good and willing people, but who have a minuscule budget, no transport, no means of communication and, sometimes, limited training and experience. It would be wonderful to sit down and get right into the whole business of AIDS prevention *per se*. More typically it is first a matter of assembling basic resources, from photocopiers to motorcycles." People with the required skills and experience are also in short supply, which means that finding personnel and training them absorbs a large proportion of the energy and attention being devoted to AIDS control work in most developing countries[5].

Not surprisingly money — how much is needed, where to get it, and how best to employ it — also absorbs a great deal of attention. National AIDS programmes have to be funded and, in the many Third World countries where annual per capita health budgets are less than the cost of a hamburger in the United States or Europe, AIDS prevention can only take place if new funding is provided. WHO has thus far organised nine international meetings (in Ethiopia, Kenya, Mozambique, Rwanda, Senegal Tanzania, Uganda, Zaire, and Zambia) at which donor countries and agencies, and the country requiring assistance, have determined the most practical ways to co-ordinate financial, material and technical aid.

'in some cases the wheels of donor bureaucracies turn slowly'

Over US$60 million has so far been pledged, though not all of this has actually arrived in the recipient countries. In some cases they draw on the pledged money as and when they need it for specific activities; in other cases the wheels of donor bureaucracies turn slowly at best, with delays of many months between a pledge and money-in-hand.

Looking ahead, Tarantola believes that "financial assistance to national programmes depends on the continued interest and commitment of the international donor community. In four or five years it could prove difficult to maintain the current momentum". Tarantola is a veteran of the successful global effort to eradicate smallpox, and knows well the extent to which such mobilisations are dependent on donor goodwill. "Our first year [in GPA] was a firefighting job, running between one request for help and another." Now, for the second year, "after a lot of thinking," they are trying to "plan what was thought a year ago to be unplannable" [6].

Though national AIDS committees are meant to take the lead on AIDS campaigns in their respective countries, a commonly-heard complaint is that "they don't seem to be doing anything beyond screening some blood, having meetings and putting up a few posters". Certainly public expectations of these committees are high, reflecting the degree of anxiety people feel about AIDS.

In reality national AIDS committees are faced with a staggering task. They must respond to a public crisis which often requires efforts on the same scale as a major disaster such as famine, flood or war. AIDS is an emergency comparable to the process of desertification, which leads to famine and which will not end this year or next. But unlike encroaching deserts the threat posed by AIDS is expanding geometrically. So the national AIDS committees must act on two fronts simultaneously: responding vigorously to contain the crisis today, while laying down the institutional framework which will sustain prevention activates for decades into the future. "It's a bit like trying to ride a galloping horse while attempting to put the saddle on and hitch up the cart at the same time", says Tarantola [7].

The "cart" in this case is a national AIDS programme which goes well beyond the health sector, informing and co-ordinating a range of responses which cut across existing sectors, departments and programmes. AIDS prevention impinges on education, economic and manpower planning, tourism promotion, transport, and even foreign affairs. It threatens the bureaucratic "turf" of many people whose jobs and goals have been far removed from health matters. But if a national AIDS programme is to work, it must be co-ordinated across the separate fiefdoms which make up the national administration. For this reason, in a number of the hardest-hit countries, national committees meet frequently, and are headed by a full-time manager who often has a direct

Governments wake up to AIDS

Since 1986 WHO's Global Programme on AIDS has recognised that the willingness of governments to initiate and support national AIDS programmes will vary and may change rapidly. Nearly every government faced with AIDS has taken more time than it should to get to grips with the epidemic, while the international press has often focused on the slowness of African governments. "Africa has been as quick to start preventive action as countries in other parts of the world," counters Dr Mann, who cites a variety of logistical and political factors which affect reporting of AIDS in any part of the world, and particularly in developing countries with overloaded health systems [11].

Collecting accurate global statistics on AIDS is hampered by lack of reporting and widespread under-recognition and diagnosis of AIDS. But, says Dr James Chin, head of GPA's AIDS surveillance, forecasting and impact assessment unit, reporting is becoming "increasingly more open and frank". Formerly chief of infectious diseases for California, Chin points to a "remarkable positive change in attitude" among Eastern Mediterranean countries which recently resulted in the establishment of national AIDS committees in 13 of 23 countries [12].

For GPA director Mann, (who before moving to WHO spent two years developing "Project SIDA", the internationally-supported official AIDS research programme in Zaire); a "watershed event" in government attitudes to AIDS was the January 1988 world summit of health ministers held in London. This meeting, attended by 140 delegations, including 117 ministers, was the first global gathering of health ministers ever to discuss a single disease. The ministers endorsed a declaration outlining measures which all should adopt in order to stop transmission of HIV, and stated that prevention programmes must respect human rights. "There are differences [among countries] but this is an extraordinary consensus," commented Dr Mann. "Now it is a matter of translating that consensus into reality." [13]

WHO staff believe that the global climate of opinion on AIDS is changing in the direction of greater candour as more countries realise that there is little to be gained by concealment. Fostering this openness and exchange is an important aspect of AIDS prevention, and one of the most important tasks of the global programme on AIDS.

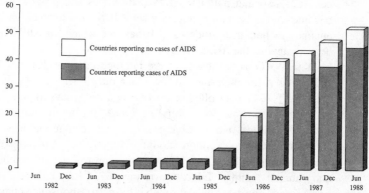

Figure 8.2 It was not until 1986 that most African countries started reporting on AIDS to the World Health Organization. By June 1988, except for Namibia and Western Sahara, every country or territory in Africa was doing so. Source: WHO

line of communication with the president or prime minister.

Initially concentrated within ministries of health, national AIDS programmes in many countries are now opening out to include people from other ministries and from non-medical disciplines. WHO encourages the national committees to set up true public health programmes which go well beyond health ministries and which include NGOs (non-governmental organisations). WHO also supports the decentralisation of responsibility for AIDS both vertically within ministries, and across sectors and disciplines. "What is still lacking", Tarantola comments, "is a sense that real authority for activities has been delegated from governments to the NGOs [such as Red Cross societies] which are represented on the national committees. At present the NGOs are consulted, and governments often like to use them to deliver programmes, but governments are slow to hand over formal authority and resources. WHO wants to speed the process along [8]."

From Dr Halfdan Mahler through Dr Jonathan Mann downwards, WHO personnel involved in the Global Programme on AIDS have constantly stressed the dangers presented by bureaucratic bottlenecks at every level. "We must always remember", Mahler told the UN General Assembly in October 1987, "that AIDS has stolen a march on us, for it spread silently and widely before we even knew of its existence or cause" [9]. By nature of what they must achieve, AIDS programmes must be innovative and draw on the resources of the whole community. "I can't say there is a cause and effect relationship", says Dr Tarantola, "but I have observed that in many countries where national AIDS committees have been broadened to include a better cross-section of the community, innovations, particularly in the field of AIDS information and education, seem to spring up" [10].

Ideally, news of successful innovations will be passed between countries, so that national AIDS committees and programmes will become true pulse points not only for AIDS surveillance, but for the changes in human attitudes and behaviour which are still our best defence against the AIDS virus.

With WHO as the leader of the international mobilisation against AIDS, what are the principles on which the global strategy is based? "If AIDS is to be controlled in any one country," says Mann, "it must be controlled in every country". Successful mobilisation requires sustained political and social commitment at the national level, where AIDS control and prevention should preferably be knitted into existing health systems and tied to a philosophy of protecting both public health and human rights. Education is the key, GPA staff believe: HIV transmission can be slowed through informed, responsible behaviour on the part of millions of individuals the world over.

WHO in the world's bedrooms

Don't be surprised if, in the near future, a polite lady or gentleman asks you how you choose your girlfriends — or boyfriends. Men and women aged 18 to 49 in dozens of countries will soon be interviewed about how they make love, how often and with whom, and how far they will travel to meet partners. The results of the WHO survey will help national AIDS programmes target education programmes by identifying changes in patterns of sexuality.

The questionnaire has been written by a group of experts from developing and developed countries in collaboration with the GPA Social and Behavioural Research (SBR) unit. The questionnaire will be adapted to reflect country and cultural sensitivities a,nd carefully selected teams will conduct personal interviews, in order to obtain a high response rate. Interviews will be complemented by a set of simultaneous analyses of specific cultures, so that the answers can be understood in their proper context.

Dr Manuel Carballo, head of SBR, hopes that the survey will elicit important data on the frequency of sexual partner change, on the age at which sexual activity begins, on what determines high-risk sexual behaviour and condom use, and on patterns of geographic mobility — all of which may vary from one country or culture to another. "By understanding the complexities of sexual behaviour we hope to become more sensitive to the needs of particular groups and provide them with information that is relevant and acceptable", Carballo explains [14].

The study is already in progress — the first wave of surveys will be conducted in Australia, Brazil, Britain, Kenya, Tanzania, Thailand, Uganda and Zambia and several European countries — and will add more countries as it goes along.

There has been little systematic study of human sexual behaviour since the 1948 and 1953 Kinsey reports on male and female sexuality in the United States. Kinsey's reports, which shocked the nation at the time of their publication, found that 18% of males were bi-sexual for at least three years between the ages of 16 and 55, and an additional 13% tended to be more homosexual than heterosexual. WHO's survey may make equally surprising discoveries — discoveries which will be indispensable for successful AIDS education around the world.

What will WHO's Global Programme on AIDS be doing in 1988-89, its second year of operation? Ongoing and planned activities include:

- Further development and strengthening of *national AIDS programmes*, helping put 78 short-term and 50 medium-term plans into effect, and holding more than a dozen donor meetings in African countries.
- Developing *evaluation strategies*, so that lessons are learned systematically from the worldwide AIDS effort.
- Collaborating with the World Bank on research into the *economic impact* of AIDS and making operational a WHO computer databank on AIDS epidemiology, serology, and impact assessment, for use by governments and academic institutions.

- Producing *guidelines* on AIDS information / education campaigns for decision-makers and educators, and guidelines on the ethical issues involved in AIDS drug and vaccine testing for science and industry AIDS policies for the workplace.
- Issuing regular information to the *media* in the form of a "Global Facts File", and preparing for World AIDS Day on 1 December 1988.
- Conducting cross-cultural surveys investigating *sexual behaviour*, intravenous drug use and how people are coping with AIDS (See Box: "WHO in the world's bedrooms").
- Organising *regional* meetings in Asia, Africa and the Americas.

Asking the right questions

Because the behaviours involved in AIDS transmission are private, often hidden, or disapproved of by many societies, AIDS educators need to know more about them in order to persuade people to modify or change their behaviour. This means learning what motivates people to engage in risky activities, especially activities involving unprotected sex and intravenous drug use; and discovering the best means of convincing them to avoid risks, and of sustaining changed attitudes and behaviour over the long-term. At present, AIDS educators have too little information about these things to design and implement effective programmes. So WHO is setting out to find answers — by asking people who are at risk what they do and why they do it.

The GPA's Social and Behavioural Research Unit is designing cross-cultural studies to investigate sexuality, drug use and the way people cope with AIDS. The drug injection study — to be carried out in urban areas, primarily in industrialised countries in summer 1988 — will yield standardised information which can be used to compare the behaviour of drug users in different countries. The surveys will identify high risk behaviours in their specific social and cultural settings, and highlight groups which need specialised education and intervention. Dr Manuel Carballo, who leads this WHO unit, believes these ongoing studies will prove immensely useful for AIDS education planners. His 10 years in charge of WHO's infant and child nutrition programmes have reinforced a conviction that durable health programmes grow from an active understanding of social and cultural realities.

"There is evidence already of short-term behaviour changes among small groups of people at high risk of AIDS", comments Belgian sociologist, Dr Michel Caraël, who works with the unit. "But we are very far from understanding how to educate entire populations about *'one of the* AIDS, and to engender behaviour changes which last." Dr Caraël *thorniest* stresses that we still know very little about what motivates people in *issues WHO* matters of health and risk. "Even the short-term changes may have been *must* motivated as much or more by the individual's perception of AIDS, *confront.'* gained from many experiences, than by information campaigns." [15]

Co-ordinating global AIDS research

WHO's Global Programme on AIDS provides a international forum for the exchange of technical and scientific information, and facilitates the development and improvement of diagnostic reagents, antiviral agents and vaccines — guiding their speedy but ethically and medically sound application to all the countries of the world. This involves discussions with scientists, research institutions, public interest groups and pharmaceutical companies.

Such discussions among the members of WHO's international expert advisory group on AIDS research have led to the recommendations that WHO should:

- Promote the *sharing of information* through meetings of international researchers and develop a database on the status of research in progress.
- Fund targeted activities in *biomedical research*, especially research that otherwise might not be carried out industrialised countries, eg: research in transmission and the diagnosis of HIV infection.

WHO itself does not intend to become a major funder of biomedical research. Rather, it sees its role as promoting research in developing countries with insufficient financial and/or technical resources, and acting as a clearing-house for the most up-to-date information and thinking on research relevant to developing countries. WHO will:

- Suggest *strategies of care* for people with AIDS in developing countries, where the high technology treatments used in North America and Europe are usually too expensive and often impractical.
- Examine *the interaction of HIV with TB*, malaria, leprosy, and other tropical diseases, and develop guidelines for managing double infections.

But these are almost routine matters compared to one of the thorniest research-related issues which WHO must confront. WHO is preparing preliminary guidelines for scientists and industry engaged in drug and vaccine testing and trials. These ethical considerations will necessarily arise when vaccines reach the stage known as "efficacy trials": critical experiments on humans to determine whether or not a *'raises moral and scientific issues of the most serious kind'*

candidate vaccine actually gives protection from infection by HIV when the individual is exposed to the virus.

In the past, such experiments have involved inoculating one group of people with a candidate vaccine against a particular infection, and then exposing this group, and an uninoculated control group, to the disease-causing bacteria or virus. Intentional exposure of *any* person, whether inoculated or not, to the AIDS virus is obviously a step which raises moral and scientific issues of the most serious kind. Yet if the effectiveness of an AIDS vaccine is to be truly tested, there seems no way around the fact that some groups will have to be vaccinated while others are not, in an environment where exposure to the AIDS virus is occurring. To be statistically sound, the groups involved in these experiments will have to be large. Ethical guidelines are thus a priority of the highest order.

Although most drugs and vaccines will be developed in industrialised countries, testing and trials are likely to be carried out in regions where HIV rates are higher. In effect this means that human trials may be more likely to take place in developing than in developed countries. The scientific reason advanced for this, particularly with vaccine trials, is that the effectiveness of the vaccine would be best demonstrated in places where rates of seroconversion — the annual numbers of people who are at present contracting the AIDS virus — are high. In regions where seroconversion rates are low it would be more difficult to detect the impact of a vaccine between those who have received it and those who have not.

The political pitfalls involved in testing a US or European-developed vaccine in the Third World are summed up in the emotive term "guinea pigs". If it were to happen, as is possible, that some people in a developing country contracted HIV while participating in vaccine trials, accusations of immoral experimentation by northern researchers would be sure to ensue. Not only must such trials be conducted ethically, according to accepted guidelines, but they must be *seen* to be ethically done. The standards of scientific and ethical behaviour required of those performing drug and vaccine tests and trials is thus very high. At stake is public confidence in the whole AIDS research enterprise, a trust which WHO views as a vital component of AIDS prevention worldwide — and is taking great care, in the drawing up of its guidelines, to protect.

Further complicating the picture is the issue of "informed consent". Will each individual involved in AIDS vaccine trials be told, and fully understand, the significance of being part of the trials? Will all participants in the trials receive information on how to protect themselves from infection (for example through using condoms), and if so, how will this affect the behaviour which leads to exposure, and thus, the outcome of the trials? If vaccines or treatments are tested in developing countries where illiteracy is prevalent, how can researchers be sure that consent has truly been "informed"?

Because Third World governments are likely to be approached by research teams from industrialised countries for permission to carry out drug and vaccine testing, WHO will ensure that any government can seek WHO advice and technical assistance should it consider permitting any of its citizens to take part in clinical trials.

'we must keep people with AIDS in society, at their job'

NGOs — what role?

Until mid-1988, most of GPA's efforts went on consultation with governments in support of national AIDS plans. However, WHO now recognises that non-governmental organisations (NGOs) are an essential part of the global mobilisation against AIDS. GPA director Dr Jonathan Mann has emphatic words for NGOs: "We are prepared to form new alliances, to build relationships with you and discuss ways of working together that may be different from what you may have done with WHO before" [16].

According to Dr Tarantola, NGOs have already played a valuable role in a number of developing countries including Kenya, Mozambique, Rwanda and Tanzania. However, many NGOs "are overstretched because they are used too much in a delivery capacity, and too little in a consultative capacity". One burden which NGOs in many countries will increasingly have to shoulder, Tarantola believes, is caring for and counselling people sick with AIDS and their families — "something governments will find very difficult to do" [17].

Another role which WHO sees for NGOs concerns the humanitarian issues which surround AIDS — among them discrimination or ostracism of people who are HIV-positive or who have AIDS. Isolation and exclusion create danger (of polarising society in a manner which drives people affected by HIV and AIDS underground); inclusion creates safety, believes WHO. "What we are talking about is not dividing the world into 'them' and 'us', but realising that we must keep people with HIV and AIDS in society, at their job, and that their identity must be protected and kept confidential" [18].

WHO in the regions

WHO's headquarters in Geneva, and the Global Programme on AIDS staff based there, are the battle-command of the organisation's co-ordinated assault on HIV. But the battlefield is global, and the ultimate success of the GPA depends on the extent to which regional and national AIDS prevention activities transform WHO's

'ministers
discussed the
AIDS issues
confronting
Islamic
societies'

international strategy from a masterplan to a reality.

A substantial part of the action required in the regions is good communication, and this has most visibly involved a series of important "gatherings of the troops" in the war on AIDS. For example, WHO regional offices in Africa have co-ordinated meetings on urgent topics such as the development of laboratory services in remote areas; of alternative HIV testing methods; and on counselling HIV-infected persons and their families. In October 1988, a major international conference on AIDS in Africa is to be held, for the first time, inside Africa: in Tanzania.

In the Asian and Pacific regions the First International Conference on AIDS and Other STDs in Asia, held in the Philippines in November 1987, attracted 500 participants who wrestled with the impact of AIDS in a region where the prevalence of HIV is so far relatively low — but under-reporting of AIDS, government overreaction to the threat, and reluctance to talk openly about sexual behaviour remain problems. At the key First International Arab Conference on AIDS, held in Cairo, Egypt in March 1988, participants including several government ministers discussed both the scientific and social AIDS issues currently confronting Islamic societies. The occasion marked the first official regional recognition that these societies are no less at risk from HIV than are societies elsewhere.

Some of the earliest and most impressive regional activity has taken place in the Americas, spearheaded by WHO's regional office (the Pan American Health Organization, known as PAHO), based in Washington DC. Supported by WHO in Geneva, PAHO organised a unique "electronic" conference on AIDS in Quito, Ecuador in September 1987. Proceedings were broadcast by satellite to over 650 locations in 30 American countries, enabling over 50,000 health workers in the region to "attend" by watching television.

The most innovative aspect of the conference was a telephone link-up which allowed some viewers to ask questions of the panel of speakers, making it the largest medical conference in world history. Commented Dr Ronald St John, co-ordinator of PAHO's Health Situation and Trends Assessment Programme: "For the first time the rank-and-file health worker who we count on to implement these [health] initiatives got to hear the information first hand, and to see the faces that went with the voices" [19]. The conference had a big impact, and a repeat performance — to be broadcast from São Paulo in September 1988 — will reach an even wider audience.

PAHO started informal surveillance of AIDS cases in 1983. At that time PAHO convened a meeting with representatives from countries which were reporting AIDS cases, and by December 1985

WHO consensus statements

WHO has issued over 30 consensus statements, reports and guidelines on AIDS. Each has been drawn up by an international group of experts. They cover many controversial issues, such as breastfeeding, immunisation, condoms and prisons. Some of the issues are:

Breastfeeding and HIV infection:
• Breastfeeding should be promoted and protected in all countries.
• HIV-infected mothers should not be discouraged from breastfeeding. Infection through nursing represents only a small, incremental risk to the infant and is far outweighed by the benefits of breastmilk [23].

HIV and child immunisation:
• Childhood immunisations are recommended for HIV-infected infants and children, except those with clinical manifestations of AIDS [24].

AIDS in prison:
• WHO recommends governments and prison authorities consider distribution of condoms, and rehabilitation programmes for intravenous drug users.
• Prisoners have the same rights of confidentiality and counselling as others.
• Prisoners with AIDS should be shown compassion, and allowed early release to "die in dignity and freedom" [25].

HIV "dementia":
• There is no evidence that otherwise healthy HIV-infected people suffer mental disturbances.
• There is no justification for HIV screening as a strategy for detecting functional impairments in otherwise healthy key workers like airline pilots, bus drivers, or staff at nuclear power stations [26].

Social aspects of AIDS:
• There is no public health rationale to justify isolation, quarantine, or any discriminatory measures based solely on the fact that a person is suspected or known to be HIV-infected.
• The avoidance of discrimination is important for AIDS prevention and control; failure to prevent discrimination may endanger public health [27].

Intravenous drug users:
• WHO will develop and co-ordinate monitoring and evaluating strategies.
• Given their economic, legal, social and epidemiological situations countries should:
— expand availability of drug treatment services;
— expand range of treatment methods;
— where feasible, make available sterile needles and syringes through distribution programmes [28].

Screening and testing:
• Screening for HIV prevents transmission through blood supplies and yields epidemiological information.
• Serosurveys must involve informed consent, confidentiality and counselling, or be anonymous.
• Voluntary testing must involve informed consent, confidentiality and counselling [29].

Screening travellers:
• Screening travellers or demanding proof of seronegativity will not prevent the spread of AIDS [30].

AIDS and the newborn:
• Voluntary testing of pregnant women with "high-risk" behaviours must be accompanied by counselling and support [31].

'selling blood is a valued income for many impoverished people' had drafted guidelines which have been updated annually. PAHO expects that by August 1988 every country in the region will have a national plan of action ready for implementation and will have received initial financial and technical assistance from GPA through PAHO. PAHO is already assisting AIDS programmes in Argentina, Brazil, Chile, Dominican Republic, Ecuador, Haiti and Mexico,

Dr Fernando Zacarias, a Mexican national who is an advisor on AIDS, believes that prevention programmes have already yielded partial successes, despite the lack of adequate scientific knowledge of sexual behaviour in the Americas. The experience of family planning associations has been invaluable.

One of PAHO's goals is to have instituted screening in public sector blood banks in all member states by the end of 1988, and in privately-run blood banks by 1989. In the absence of screening the Mexican Government has forbidden private blood banks to operate, and donors are no longer paid for giving blood. Repeated selling of blood at different blood banks is a valued source of income for many impoverished people — people whose other activities, such as drug use or prostitution, may increase their chances of contracting HIV and of passing it on through their blood donations. PAHO has organised training workshops in Brazil Mexico, and Puerto Rico and has received requests from Costa Rica El Salvador, Guatemala, Honduras, Nicaragua, and Panama, for assistance in blood screening.

PAHO member states have some of the highest national per capita AIDS case totals in the world, and the organisation is urgently examining the epidemiology of HIV in the region. "But is is also extremely important", says Dr Zacarias, "for us to find out how HIV infection interacts with other diseases, such as leprosy and leishmaniasis, which are common in the region" [20]. Future plans include behavioural research and possibly drug and vaccine trials. Both St John and Zacarias are acutely conscious of the load which HIV and AIDS are now putting on health systems which are already stretched to the breaking point. "A number of cities in Latin America are growing faster, and will soon be larger, than almost any other part of the world," says St John, "and health services must be provided for these internal immigrants who suffer not only from the communicable diseases of the under-developed world, but also from the 'modern' urban diseases brought on by factors such as environmental pollution and stress" [21].

Most of Latin America's population over the next decades will be under 15 years of age: a huge group in urgent need of AIDS education before sexual activity begins. And this must be undertaken in the midst of, as Dr Zacarias puts it, "a persistent regional economic crisis which will probably get worse before it gets better".

Nevertheless Zacarias, like many of his colleagues, remains

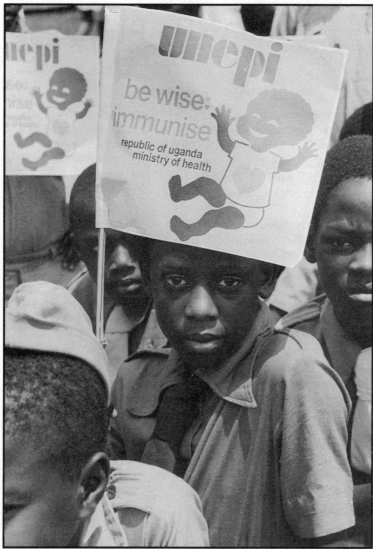

SCF/ Penny Tweedie

Figure 8.3
There is no evidence that child immunisation campaigns have been spreading the AIDS virus. WHO and UNICEF are helping developing countries to ensure that re-usable needles are properly sterilised, and that a cheap one-time needle that cannot be re-used is being developed.

cautiously optimistic: "In the countries of the region, everybody wants to do something", he commented, "and people are concerned that they are not doing enough — I think that's a very healthy attitude" [22].

CHAPTER NINE

HUMANITARIAN ISSUES

Whether we like it or not, AIDS has arrived on our planet. Each affected group, each community and country, is having to wrestle with the problems of AIDS in its own way. Each tackles AIDS in the context of its own history, traditions, legal system — and internal conflicts. Each will find different answers, and strike different balances between the rights and needs of individuals, of minority groups and those of society as a whole.

Governments and other responsible bodies have a duty to show leadership in the protection of their societies from AIDS. This duty has been interpreted both inside and outside of governments in two broadly different — and predictable — ways.

Because of the way the virus spreads, and the consequent fact that AIDS attacks some groups before others, some argue that the protection of society at large entails taking measures *against* groups or individuals affected by AIDS. For those who define the problem in this way, medical and legal measures which create distance between people with HIV and AIDS, or those defined as likely to contract HIV or AIDS, and society in general, are seen as solutions. At their most extreme these "separatist" solutions involve the imposition of quarantine on all people with HIV and AIDS.

Others argue that, while some groups have been affected by AIDS before others, the epidemic is one which confronts society as a whole, not just the parts of it which have been affected first. From this point of view the enemy is not other people, but the AIDS virus, and the duty to protect society is thus a duty to protect all its members. The biggest danger, according those who define the problem in this way, is the tendency to divide society into those who are, or might be, infected, and those who are not. To allow this to happen, they say, is to allow the AIDS virus to divide and rule.

Which approach is best? Heated debate on this question continues in almost every country where AIDS or HIV has appeared. There is no universal solution. No single model of social response to the epidemic appears suitable for all. Although AIDS has often aroused the deep compassion and care that human beings are capable of giving to each other, it has also, like plague, syphilis and other epidemics before it, given rise to hostility, anger and, above all, fear. People with AIDS or HIV, or suspected to be ill or carrying the virus, have been subject to social or economic discrimination and, not infrequently, violent attack. Sometimes the response to AIDS has been political and manipulated, dangerous not just for those victimised but for society as a whole.

Yet there is a yardstick available which can be used as a guide toward the types of policies and measures which are needed. The yardstick is a pragmatic one, and it asks the question: which responses to HIV and AIDS are most likely, over the long run, to succeed in containing the AIDS pandemic by preventing further infections? Given that we are in the very early stages of a global epidemic which is likely to last many decades, the evaluation of responses according to their likely long-term effect in containing HIV is important.

'in a climate of fear and blame many important options cannot be discussed'

The pragmatic yardstick encompasses the notion that a key factor in society's response to AIDS is the general level of knowledge and climate of public opinion in which decisions and policies are shaped. A climate of factually-grounded confidence is one which is most likely to engender successful policies. Conversely, in a climate of fear and blame many potentially important policy options cannot even be discussed.

This chapter looks at some of the humanitarian issues that have arisen since AIDS was first diagnosed. These issues are seldom clear-cut, for at their heart lie basic questions about the rights and responsibilities of individuals towards their community and of the state towards individuals. Where possible the issues are illustrated with examples from around the world. These are not representative, nor are they meant to single out or blame any particular country. Their purpose is simply to demonstrate that behind the philosophical debate human lives are involved.

"High-risk groups": a misleading label

Many health authorities have designated groups such as homosexual men, Haitians, Africans, prostitutes, intravenous drug users or haemophiliacs as "high-risk groups". The implication — to which this designation appears to give official sanction — is that all individuals belonging to such groups are equally likely to contract the virus and to pass it on. As a result, members of such groups have often been the targets for social isolation or worse.

A frequent focus for such attacks has been homosexuals. In 1986 one Brazilian doctor wrote that "if AIDS is limited to homosexuals, it will be a disease of public service" [1]. The following year, in a letter to the Soviet Academy of Medical Sciences, students in Moscow wrote that AIDS was "a noble epidemic" which will "wipe out all drug addicts, homosexuals and prostitutes"[2]. Also in 1987 the Washington DC Spanish language paper *La Prensa* asked: "Should society help these people who are marked by death to escape victorious from their disease? .... Should a taxpayer pay for the cure of someone who has been the victim *'what matters is what you do, not who you are'* of the use, abuse and degeneration of their sexual organs? .... Readers should judge for themselves and come to their own conclusions." [3]

Chapter Six of this dossier pointed out the effect of the categorisation of Haitians as a "high-risk group" by the US Centers for Disease Control: high unemployment, attacks on children, failed businesses and evictions. Africans in the Soviet Union have had "AIDS" shouted at them in the street [4], while Africans in India were shunned when newspapers revealed that some students from Africa had tested positive for HIV antibodies [5]. Prostitutes complain that they are accused of spreading AIDS, although in many cases they report that their clients offer to pay more for sex without condoms [6].

A further implication of this categorisation into "high-risk groups" is to suggest that anyone who does *not* belong to one of these groups is safe — and that AIDS only hits defined groups to which the majority of people do not belong. From this vantage point a seronegative, monogamous homosexual couple is erroneously labelled as more at risk of AIDS than a heterosexual man who sleeps with many partners and eventually encounters one who has already been infected with HIV. Similarly, the tendency to categorise people in this way does not take into account the fact that an intravenous drug user who does not share needles is at no greater risk from HIV than the non-drug user.

The saying "what matters is what you do, not who you are" reveals the fallacy which has arisen from repeated use of the term "high-risk group" to designate those most affected by AIDS in the earlier stages of the pandemic. More and more, public health officials talk of "high-risk activities" rather than "high-risk groups".

Ostracism, discrimination and attack

Many individuals and organisations point to growing evidence that people with HIV or AIDS, and their families and friends, are subject to discrimination and attack.

Homosexuals in countries around the world have been documented as frequent targets. One monitoring group in the United States reported 7,008 incidents of abuse and violence in 1987, a rise of 40% on the previous year. These incidents included 64 homicides — and in 15% of all cases the aggressors referred to AIDS [7]. In San Francisco another group reported that not only were attacks on homosexuals increasing, but they were becoming more violent [8]. In Brazil a wave of murders of homosexual men and *travestis* (transvestites) [9] has been attributed to fear of AIDS. Up to 300 have been murdered in the last three years and a team of detectives has been appointed to investigate crimes of violence against homosexual men [10]. There have been similar reports from Mexico [11].

In 1987 a British nurse who contracted HIV after being accidentally pierced with a contaminated syringe "became the target of a vicious hate campaign" of anonymous letters to her employers [12]. In Norway a 30-year-old barman was fired by his employer for being HIV-positive, but both the lower and middle courts supported the barman's right to retain his job. Holidaying in Tunisia to escape the pressure of his court battles, he was recognised by Norwegian compatriots who, together with other guests at his hotel, demanded that he be ejected [13].

In the Philippines a young "hospitality woman" who returned to her home town to deliver her baby was isolated in a hospital storage room which displayed the sign "Beware, AIDS patient"[14]. Refusal to treat, serve or assist people known or thought to carry HIV has been a very common reaction to the AIDS epidemic, with instances occurring in virtually every country where the virus has surfaced. Private hospitals in

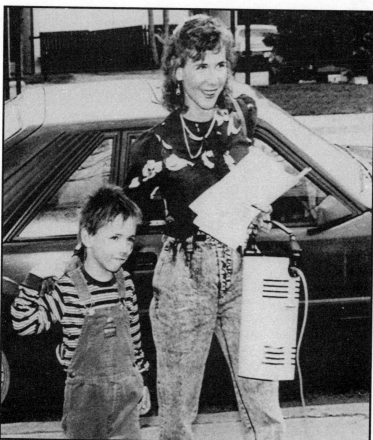

Figure 9.1
Five-year-old Jonathan contracted AIDS from a blood transfusion just after birth. His dream was to attend school before he died, instead of being taught privately at home, and his mother fought school officials in Colorado, US, until they agreed. Jonathan told his classmates: "I have a disease. My bad blood could kill you." Pictured after his first day at school, Jonathan was asked if it was fun. "Yeah, they listened and they played with me."

Ed Andrieski/ AP

'Fear is a common and powerful factor.'

Brazil have denied treatment to AIDS patients, and in a publicised case of refusal by one Catholic hospital several such patients died as a result. The hospital was taken to court but the charges were dismissed [15].

Children with HIV or AIDS, usually acquired as a result of blood transfusion treatments for haemophilia, have been subjected to abuse in several countries, including the United Kingdom and the United States. In the US state of Florida the three HIV-positive sons of a haemophiliac family were barred from attending class by school authorities, and their house was burned by arsonists. In contrast to the treatment they had received, however, they were given a warm welcome by the community and school of the town to which they then moved [16].

AIDS and the workplace

In institutionalised settings the question of AIDS becomes more complex. In the workplace more and more employers are discovering that they have workers who are HIV-positive or who have fallen ill with AIDS. There are a number of priorities which appear to come into conflict in such a situation. These include the need to maintain good relations among the staff, the wish and legal right of the employee to continue working, and the aim of management to reduce unnecessary costs.

Fear is a common and powerful factor. A 1988 US poll of employee opinions on HIV in the workplace found that 65% of those interviewed "would be concerned about using the same bathroom as an AIDS sufferer on the job, 40% were concerned about using the same cafeteria, and 37% said they would not be willing to use the same equipment" [17]. Police, firefighters and paramedics were more fearful than other employees, believing in some cases that "a policeman should be able to use any force necessary to prevent his contracting AIDS, [which in extreme cases] might mean shooting a person known to have AIDS who was trying to bite an officer" [18]. A March 1987 poll of over 300 companies in the United Kingdom revealed that 20% would ask people with AIDS to resign and 4% would ignore official guidelines not to dismiss them [19].

The ungrounded fear of casual infection often spreads beyond the workplace. In Canada lack of confidentiality regarding testing resulted in a teacher being transferred to a non-teaching post at the insistence of parents afraid of infection [20]. In France the authorities refused to accredit a probationary teacher after he informed them he had AIDS; in this case, however, he returned to work when parents, colleagues and pupils demonstrated their strong support for him [21].

A number of companies have decided to screen potential employees before offering them work. In Spain in 1987 applicants for 1,000 new jobs at a General Motors plant were reportedly being tested by the company [22], while in Paris in early 1988 the municipal government had apparently been testing probationary employees for HIV without their consent [23]. At the same time the British subsidiary of the transnational oil company, Texaco, introduced compulsory HIV-antibody tests for potential new employees [24]. The airlines British Airways, Lufthansa and SAS all screen either potential pilots or all new employees [25].

'Not every company has seen AIDS as a threat'

The issue of AIDS or HIV in the workplace is not restricted to particular companies or even particular governments. It has been reported that US State Department medical personnel travelled to Africa in late 1986, in part to calm fears current among US employees there as to "whether the [AIDS] virus could be caught from insects or from food prepared by a local cook, and whether [African] nationals working in embassies and residences should be tested for AIDS" [26]. Several countries, notably South Africa and Middle Eastern countries, which rely on very large numbers of foreign workers, require those applying for work permits to be tested for antibodies to HIV in their country of origin, and reject any who test positive. No member of the US armed forces can be transferred overseas if he or she is carrying the virus.

Not every country and not every company has seen AIDS or HIV as a threat to employers or employees. In 1986 in Uganda, Barclays Bank issued guidelines that employees with AIDS were to be guaranteed the same rights as all other employees and were entitled to the same sickness benefits [27]. In the United States a growing number of companies have policy guidelines for dealing with AIDS in the workplace, although different studies give estimates ranging from 10% [28] to 29% [29] of corporations. The question of AIDS in the workplace has been described as not a problem with patients, but with those around them "who are reacting to the general panic over AIDS" [30].

In March 1988 the US federal Office of Personnel Management (OPM) issued guidelines to federal agencies on dealing with issues related to AIDS and the workplace, including education, the right to work, confidentiality and employee concerns. The OPM recommends that managers recognise the fears of co-workers, provide education and information, and be sensitive to the right of an employee who is HIV-positive, or has AIDS, to work as long as medically possible. It recommends that disciplinary procedures be eventually taken if co-workers refuse to co-operate [31].

In the United Kingdom fewer companies have issued guidelines. A circular issued by the government in 1986 stated that employees have statutory rights against dismissal "which are not reduced in any way just because an individual is infected [with HIV]" [32]. British Rail, the state-run railway network, advised workers in 1987 that the first reaction to a colleague with HIV should be of care and consideration, and it has emphasised that there is no risk of infection in normal circumstances [33]. In the same year a cinema projectionist, homosexual but not known to be

'reports of
individual
nurses and
doctors
refusing
treatment'

HIV-positive, was dismissed on the grounds that his life-style posed a risk to fellow employees. Although an employment tribunal initially found in favour of his employers, a higher court eventually ruled that he had been unfairly dismissed and was entitled to compensation [34]. A similar case in West Germany, of a clerk who was seropositive, ended with the ruling that the employer was guilty of neglecting his responsibilities towards the employee [35].

The reactions of health workers

In many countries health and other social workers, such as fire and rescue brigades, whose jobs might bring them into close bodily contact with perons with HIV or AIDS, have expressed fears that they might accidentally contract the virus. The example of Brazil, given above, is not the only country where patients with AIDS or HIV have been refused treatment by hospital staff on account of such fears. In China, when a US citizen with AIDS fell ill, he was left unattended and in isolation, because medical personnel had no experience of the syndrome and feared infection [36].

There have been scattered reports from many other countries in Europe, Asia, the Americas and Africa of individual nurses and sometimes doctors refusing treatment. Anxiety has been compounded by hospitals which have refused treatment to AIDS patients for financial or administrative reasons. In the United States in 1983 a sick man was flown from Florida to San Francisco because the Florida state authorities did not wish to bear the costs of caring for him [37].

Despite such reports, the response of health professionals has, in general, been to assume the responsibility of caring for all who are sick, whether or not HIV or AIDS is the cause. To reinforce this, such bodies as the British Royal College of Nursing [38], the British Medical Association [39] and the American Medical Association in the United States [40], among others, have issued policy statements saying that HIV and AIDS do not constitute grounds for refusing to care for the sick. Doctors, nurses and other health workers who refuse to treat patients on these grounds are, according to these official statements, liable to be found guilty of professional misconduct.

Cases of health workers acquiring HIV in the course of their duties are rare — worldwide only a handful have been documented in the seven years since AIDS was first diagnosed [41]. None of the documented cases involved casual contact. In each case the health worker came into contact, either by means of an unusual accident or during unprotected surgery, with quantities of HIV-contaminated blood. In each case health authorities point out that infection could have been avoided if routine precautions such as wearing protective clothing or observing proper laboratory safeguards had been adopted. (Some commentators have observed that carelessness on the part of research laboratory workers is still all too common, despite widespread publicity about the need for scrupulous laboratory practice in the age of AIDS [42].)

'consultants called for the right to test patients secretly'

Official reassurances notwithstanding, a proportion of doctors still express fear of treating patients with HIV or AIDS. In the United States some opinion polls of hospital residents and medical students have recorded that a substantial minority feel that they would be justified in refusing to treat such patients [43]. And in Britain in June 1988 a number of consultants called for the right to test patients secretly if they were suspected of being seropositive. BMA officials have stated that such testing would be not only unethical, but possibly also illegal [44].

The extremist fringe

Extremist groups in some Western countries, notably the United States and France, have been quick to exploit AIDS. Mostly their targets have been blacks and homosexual men.

In 1987 the *Thunderbolt*, a broadsheet published by an obscure "white power" group in Georgia, argued that AIDS comes from Africa and is endangering the white race through black bisexual men in the United States. Blacks are "genetically prone to AIDS" and black men are infecting white women who are "victims of race-mixing" it said [45]. Another obscure group, the Christian Defense League, claimed in 1987 that "whites who have debased themselves by having sex with ... colored carriers risk becoming gravely ill. ... White homosexuals could have started their race's exposure to AIDS by seeking out colored sexual partners ... Regardless, whites in the beginning got AIDS from colored." [46]

The French political party, the National Front, which believes that France is being "swamped" by African immigrants, has found AIDS a useful extra argument. In July 1987, a magazine associated with the Front explained that AIDS started in Africa when a black man sodomised a monkey — a supposedly essential fact that the author claimed was being suppressed by the French health authorities [47]. At a National Front rally in the lead up to the 1988 presidential election (in which its candidate, Jean-Marie Le Pen, received 14% of the vote), the ballad of Joan of Arc was rewritten to include the words "Oh Joan, if you could see the France you loved, riddled with drugs and AIDS..." [48].

The Nebraska-based Family Research Institute, which considers that "of all the vices, only homosexuality constitutes a conspiracy against society" [49], claimed in 1987 that because of the "promiscuity and incredibly unsanitary sexual practices [of homosexuals], pathogens once localised in a given geographic region are rapidly being spread

'teenage throughout the world. AIDS is a first fruit of this process and more
inmates plagues stemming from homosexual behavior are bound to occur." [50]
could apply The anti-Jewish views of a minority of black Muslims were reinforced
for condoms' by the remarks of a black aide to the mayor of Chicago, to followers of
the black Muslim leader Louis Farrakhan. In 1988 this aide reportedly
claimed that "Jewish doctors were injecting black babies with the AIDS
virus" [51].

Prisons: transmission risks magnified

Prison authorities the world over are discovering not only that more and
more of their inmates are ill with AIDS or carrying HIV, but that the
prison environment itself is conducive to spreading the virus. Single-sex
prisons lead to homosexual encounters, both voluntary and forced, while
the presence of drugs, together with contraband needles and no means of
sterilisation, leads to rapid transmission through intravenous drug use.
The following description could have come from a number of countries
on any continent.

"In Osasco [prison], 50, [or] 70 inmates used one syringe. It came to you
with drops of blood from the last man who'd used it. We knew the risks,
but what could we do?" said L.R. in a prison hospital in São Paulo, Brazil,
in early 1987, when he was already suffering severe weight loss from
AIDS [52].

When prisoners have been screened for HIV they often show a far higher
rate of infection than in the general population. In the canton of Berne,
Switzerland, 11% of inmates were reported seropositive in 1987 [53]; in
the same year the figure for new prisoners was reported as 16.8% in Italy
and 26% in Spain [54], while the average figure for France, including
smaller provincial prisons, was reckoned to be 6% in 1988 [55].

The response of authorities to the AIDS epidemic in their prisons has
varied from country to country. By the end of 1987 six countries in
Europe were distributing condoms to inmates [56], but the same measure
had been rejected in other countries, including Britain, on the grounds
that to do so would be seen as condoning homosexuality, which, although
practised, is illegal in British jails [57]. Only one US state, Vermont, was
distributing condoms [58], while in Ontario, Canada, teenage inmates
could apply for condoms, but adults could not [59]. The question of
distribution of needles or sterilising equipment was more controversial;
no authority had reported supplying its prisoners with such equipment by
mid-1988.

The question of whether or not to isolate prisoners with HIV or AIDS
has also been debated; isolation units have been reported from such places
as Dublin [60], São Paulo [61] and New York [62]. In 1987 there were riots
in Belgium by prisoners who believed themselves at risk, demanding that

HIV-positive inmates be kept apart [63].

Where isolation has occurred, however, the results have not always been beneficial. The isolation wing on Riker's Island, one of New York's prisons, was described in early 1988 as being filthy, unattended and littered with excrement [64]. Nor has the treatment offered prisoners who fall ill with AIDS always been humane. Again in New York, in 1986, 812 prisoners with AIDS, both men and women, were shackled to their beds in public hospitals with armed guards placed at their door. About 30 prisoners, six of them women, are known to have died in chains [65].

In Thailand over 40 prisoners with AIDS or HIV, some of whom became infected after being imprisoned, have reportedly been refused medical treatment [66]. Many of them are foreign and hopes were raised in 1987 that they would benefit from the general pardon issued to prisoners to celebrate the King's birthday. They were not included, however, because, according to a government spokesman, their offences involved drug-trafficking. In early 1988 one or two were reported to be very ill and not expected to survive [67].

In Brazil in early 1987, newspapers carried interviews with a number of prisoners who begged to be allowed home to die. One of them, D., was quoted as saying: "I know I'm going to die and I'm not afraid. But for the love of God let me be pardoned so that I can spend my last days with my family. They know I've got AIDS... and they don't reject me as [the prisoners] do here." [68] As a result, the authorities were preparing to forward such applications for pardon to the appeal court.

HIV and AIDS faces both jailers and prisoners with seemingly intractable problems. Prisons in most parts of the world are already overcrowded and underfunded. In an environment based on lack of trust, both AIDS education and responsible behaviour are made doubly difficult. Prison authorities emphasise that their difficulties have been increased by press reports which sensationalise AIDS and give credence to fears of casual transmission. In addition to Belgium (see above) prisoners in the United States [69], France and West Germany [70] have demanded to be segregated from inmates who were known or believed to have AIDS.

The issues raised by AIDS in society at large are magnified in the closed and stressful prison environment. Their successful resolution is essential for two reasons. Good public health practice requires that prisoners, like any other segment of the population, be taught how to protect themselves from HIV infection and allowed to practise what they have been taught. And prisoners, like anyone else, belong to the society to which most of them will eventually return. To allow a prison to become focus for HIV infection is to create a situation in which that infection will almost inevitably at some point be transferred to other members of society outside.

'30 prisoners are known to have died in chains'

Mandatory testing and reporting

The information below has been collected from various sources. Every effort has been made to check its accuracy. However, some countries impose restrictions by regulation rather then legislation and this may not be reported abroad. Some countries have passed laws but not enforced them, while others have imposed restrictions in practice but officially deny they are doing so. In some cases different government departments have different policies, and the foreign ministry (for example) may not be aware of what is being done by the health or another ministry.

AUSTRIA: Licensed prostitutes must take a routine blood test every six weeks. If the test proves positive for HIV-antibodies their licence is withdrawn but they are entitled to apply for a state pension [78].

BULGARIA: Bulgaria intends to test all citizens by 1990 [79].

CUBA: In a three-year programme Cuba is testing all citizens; all those discovered HIV-positive are placed in quarantine.

WEST GERMANY: In Bavaria candidates for state employment and judiciary posts must be screened for HIV antibodies. Individuals suspected of being infected with HIV (prostitutes and intravenous drug users are automatically suspected) must be screened, with the test repeated quarterly if the result is negative. Seropositive individuals "whose conduct endangers others" can be isolated [80].

GUATEMALA: Female prostitutes are reported subject to periodic tests for STDs (including antibodies to HIV) [81].

HUNGARY: The partners of individuals known to be HIV-positive, individuals on prostitution charges, individuals with or suspected of having a sexually-transmitted disease and intravenous drug users are subject to mandatory testing [82].

ICELAND: Icelandic law allows isolation of carriers of contagious life-threatening diseases, including HIV and AIDS.

IRAQ: According to the Official Gazette of 27 May 1987, all citizens returning from abroad must be tested for HIV antibodies.

ISRAEL: Prostitutes, among other groups specified by the ministry of health, are subject to six-monthly tests for HIV antibodies [83].

JAMAICA: Reportedly screens migrant farm workers before they leave Jamaica [84].

KOREA (SOUTH KOREA): Prostitutes, bar hostesses and employees of night clubs are tested every six months [85]. "High-risk" HIV carriers are to be interned. Initial government proposal to detain all seropositive individuals was successfully opposed by the Korean Medical Association [86].

PANAMA: In the district of La Chorrera and elsewhere women working in specified establishments (bars, boarding-houses, hotels, brothels and other "entertainment centres") are subject to three-monthly tests for HIV antibodies [87].

SOUTH AFRICA: According to the Government Gazette of 30 October 1987 any foreigner or citizen may be tested if required by a medical officer; deportation or isolation of those infected is legal.

SWEDEN: Law no. 1406 of 18 December 1986 allows a person with a venereal disease (including HIV infection) to be detained in hospital. At least four such cases have occurred.

SYRIA: Scholarship students returning from abroad are tested [88].

Mandatory testing and reporting (continued)

USA: Nationwide, all military service volunteers are tested. All servicemen are tested before being posted abroad; those found positive are not allowed to leave the USA on active service [89]. All immigrants and refugees are tested.most states have passed legislation regarding AIDS, some in protection of individual rights, others apparently restricting individual rights. For example, in Illinois and Louisiana marriage licence applicants must take the HIV antibody test[90]. And in New York legislation has been proposed to ensure that sexual partners of people with AIDS are informed that they

might also have been infected [91].

USSR: All citizens and foreigners are tested "where there are grounds for suspecting infection". Mandatory testing is imposed on citizens returning home after one month abroad, foreigners staying longer than three months, persons belonging to risk groups, citizens "in contact" with AIDS patients carriers, citizens and foreigners "expressing a wish" to undergo testing [92].

(For a list of restrictions relating specifically to travel or immigration see Appendix II.)

WHO considers that governments should consider condom distribution and rehabilitation programmes for drug users as part of their programmes for the prevention and control of AIDS in prisons. In addition, prisoners should have the same rights of confidentiality and counselling as all those at risk from HIV and AIDS, and governments should consider the early release of prisoners dying from AIDS (see Chapter Eight).

AIDS and quarantine

The basic right to protection from arbitrary arrest, detention and imprisonment is legally recognised in many countries with differing political systems, and by several international conventions. But most countries also have legislation which allows authorities to isolate or quarantine people suffering from highly contagious diseases. The diseases usually covered by such regulations are those in which the infection is spread by casual contact, by coughs or sneezes, by touching or through contact with personal items such as infected clothing or utensils.

AIDS does not fall into the above category because it is *not* transmitted by casual contact. In everyday situations, and with the exception of unprotected sexual intercourse, the person with HIV or AIDS does not pose a risk of infection to those around him or her. However, a number of countries, particularly those where current AIDS cases are few, have enacted legislation which specifically allows them to isolate people with HIV or AIDS.

In Cuba, which is believed to be the only country to place every individual carrying the virus in quarantine as soon as he or she is detected, the rationale is to save costs by preventing an epidemic. "Our country is a poor country". said the deputy minister of public health, Hector Terry, in 1987. "If many Cubans become infected and sick, I do not know how we would take care of them. It would cost too much. We really have to prevent such a situation." [71] By early 1988 174 individuals were known to be held in the special sanatorium in Havana [72].

In South Korea, which has discussed plans to impose mandatory isolation on members of so-called "high-risk groups", the rationale is less clear, especially since any individual who knows he or she is seropositive and who has sexual relations is subject to three years imprisonment [73]. Legislation in South Africa, the Soviet Union and the West German state of Bavaria gives authorities the power to isolate people with HIV, although the use of this power has not yet been reported.

In other countries where quarantine has been used, it has been limited to selected individuals, generally those who for one reason or another have been judged a danger to society. In Iceland an HIV-positive woman was reportedly quarantined under existing legislation on contagious diseases [74]. There have been four cases of isolation in Sweden, including that of a drug user whose friends asked for him to be taken in because, they alleged, "his actions endangered them" [75]. In India, a number of prostitutes were held until a group of their supporters took the state of Tamil Nadu to court. The court decided that the state had exceeded its powers in detaining the women, and they were subsequently freed [76]. In the United Kingdom in 1988 a member of parliament claimed: "A number of young people with the AIDS virus are being detained in order to take them out of sexual circulation" [77].

With the exception of Cuba, no country is known to be routinely practising quarantine, although this may occur secretly elsewhere. Mass quarantine was tried earlier this century to try and prevent the spread of syphilis in the United States. Medical historians record how, during the First World War, the US Congress passed legislation supporting the quarantine of prostitutes suspected of spreading the disease. More than 20,000 women were held in camps on the grounds that they were suspected of transmitting syphilis, a programme which had "no apparent impact on rates of infection" [93].

Implications and costs

The rationale behind quarantine is that it is possible to divide the world physically between those with HIV or AIDS and those without. In this way transmission of HIV could be halted. Cuba is taking this line of reasoning to its logical conclusion: the mass and repeated testing of the entire adult population. An apparently easier alternative would be to test mandatorily members of designated "high-risk groups".

Although the categorisation of "high-risk groups" fails to take into account basic facts about the transmission of HIV, its strong appeal has been shown by several public opinion polls. When asked whether people with AIDS should be quarantined, 40% of US, 30% of British and 30% of Greek respondents said yes [94]. Twenty-one per cent of French and 28% of Greek respondents thought homosexuals should be quarantined, while 25% of Norwegian, 27% of British, 29% of French and Greek, and 44% of Swedish people asked thought intravenous drug users should be isolated [95].

'28% thought homosexuals should be quarantined'

In 1986 a California state referendum defeated a measure called Proposition 64, which called for quarantine and internment of people with AIDS, their suspected associates and anyone who tested positive for HIV. The measure required that all those suspected of carrying the virus be required to report to local health authorities for testing. Anyone failing to report a person with AIDS would be fined US$1,000 and jailed for 90 days. And anyone detained under the measure would lose their automatic right to 'habeas corpus' and judicial review. Although eventually defeated, Proposition 64 received slightly over two million votes, 29% of those who voted [96].

A major difficulty with quarantine as an AIDS prevention measure is the number of people involved. If all those carrying the virus are to be isolated, facilities would have to be found for about a million people in the United States, 40,000 in Italy, 50,000 in each of Britain, Australia and Canada, 200,000 in France and five to 10 million worldwide.

Where would all these people be interned? Who would pay for their keep? A number of people carrying the virus would remain undetected because they would test negative and others would be unjustly held because they were "false-positives".

Mandatory testing of "high-risk groups" has also been proposed as a tougher response to the AIDS crisis, but there is less to the argument than meets the eye. Not only would those who are seropositive but not members of a "high-risk group" remain undetected, but such testing would only be of value if some means of separation were proposed. Quarantine is the most radical suggestion, but other tactics have been put forward, among them the carrying of HIV-free identity cards [97], the tattooing of seropositives [98] and the restriction of the rights of travel, employment and association of people with HIV.

In order to have any appreciable effect in slowing the spread of HIV, mandatory testing would need to be applied broadly. But testing is both fallible (in a relatively small percentage of cases) and costly. A recent US study concluded that a national mandatory premarital screening programme would find approximately 1,200 new cases of HIV infection, equal to 0.01% of the total number currently infected. But the margin of error in the blood tests used would mean that programme would also

*'the US
military
screening
programme
cost more
that the
annual
budget of
WHO on
AIDS '*

incorrectly identify as many as 380 virus-free individuals as being infected, and would mistakenly assure an estimated 100 HIV-carriers that they were uninfected [99].

Furthermore, it would be difficult, if not impossible, to impose testing on all those who do not want to be tested. In West Germany, many homosexual men and drug users are known to have left the state of Bavaria to avoid mandatory testing [100]. In the United States, Illinois and Louisiana passed laws in 1987 requiring all applicants for marriage licences to submit to an HIV antibody blood test before a licence could be issued. The immediate result was a fall in the numbers of people applying for marriage licences in those places — by 40% in Illinois — and a rise in the numbers crossing borders to get married in adjacent states [101].

The US military, which screens all new volunteers as well as existing personnel, spent US$43 million between 1986 and 1988 on its screening programme, testing 3.2 million people [102]. To identify the 5,890 seropositive individuals detected, the US military spent US$7,300 per person, with the likelihood that a percentage of recently infected people were not identified because they tested falsely negative, and equally that some of those who were rejected were sent away on the basis of falsely positive results. Few institutions or countries could afford a measure so expensive, particularly if it had to be sustained over years or decades.

The cost of the US military screening programme is greater than the current annual budget of the WHO global programme on AIDS. Could the equivalent resources, if spent on public education and voluntary testing, counselling and support programmes, be more effective in combating AIDS?

Experience has indicated that where such control measures such as mandatory testing are seriously considered by the authorities, the number of requests for testing by individuals who think they may have been exposed to HIV falls. Conversely, public awareness campaigns in the media result in a swelling of the numbers presenting for voluntary testing, as in Britain [103]. An atmosphere of coercion has the effect of frightening people away from testing and treatment centres, in effect driving AIDS underground.

Compassion is good prevention

Harsh measures can "boomerang", having exactly the opposite effects on AIDS control to those their advocates expect. In the words of the recently-retired WHO director-general Dr Halfdan Mahler, "AIDS shows us precisely how discrimination, marginalisation, and stigmatisation are themselves threats to public health" [104].

There is no technical solution to the AIDS epidemic: no vaccine, no cure, no practical means of separating those who have already been exposed to the virus from those who have not. The principal routes of transmission of the virus — sex and intravenous drug use — are the activities of individuals, and the daily result of millions of individual decisions taken by people in every country in the world. While the notion of coercive control of these myriad decisions is an absurdity, the possibility of influencing their outcome is not. "Individual behaviour is responsible for most HIV transmission [which] requires the active participation

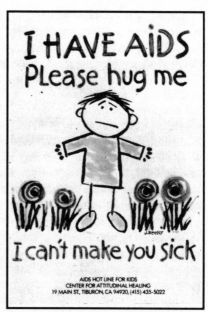

Figure 9.2
A poster from the Center for Attitudinal Healing in California. People with AIDS, adults as well as children, need affection and community contact, not isolation.

of two persons; therefore, the chain of transmission can be broken by the individual behaviour of either the infected or the non-infected person. ... the proper focus of prevention is behaviour, not infection status" [105]. Compassion, applied equally to those who have AIDS and those who do not, to those who are already infected and those who are not, makes good public health sense. It dictates that the overriding thrust of AIDS prevention must be to inform, influence and support changes in the behaviour which put people at risk. Since we cannot know everyone who already has, or who may develop, risky behaviour, everyone should be given information and education about AIDS. And experience of other disease control efforts tells us that if compassion is withdrawn from people with AIDS or HIV and they are stigmatised, fear of the disease will increase and will undermine AIDS education programmes.

Compassion is neither a "soft" nor a lax option: it is the most direct path to effective AIDS prevention.

"Although we tend to view compassion as a *feeling* between individuals, in fact, it is a much broader concept... In *societal* terms, compassion must be seen as the collective will and political acts that bring about resources, structures, institutions, behaviours, and norms directed at the care of the sick, the prevention of illness, and the promotion of health." This view was recently expressed in a prominent US medical journal [106]. A similar conclusion was reached in the report published by the Chairman of the US Presidential Commission on the Human Immunodeficiency Virus Epidemic in June 1988.

'Compassion is the most direct path to AIDS prevention'

According to this chairman's report, a key element in AIDS control is the need to prevent, at all levels of society, discrimination against people with HIV or AIDS. *"HIV-related discrimination is impairing this nation's ability to limit the spread of the epidemic* ... public health officials will not be able to gain the confidence and co-operation of infected individuals or those at high risk for infection if such individuals fear that they will be unable to retain their jobs and their housing, and that they will be unable to obtain the medical and support services they need because of discrimination based on a positive HIV antibody test." [107] The US National Academy of Sciences underlined the same message in its report in the same month: "The committee believes that fear of discrimination is a major constraint to the wide acceptance of many effective public health measures" [108].

Although the response of many societies towards the epidemic of AIDS and HIV infection has often been less than ideal, the individual response has not lacked compassion. This public response to AIDS was well-described in May 1988 in the *Journal of the American Medical Association*: "Thousands of family members and loved ones, members of voluntary community-based organisations, individuals in governmental agencies, clergy, and others and tens of thousands of health care workers have faced the panic and their own personal discomfort and fears head-on and have exemplified the very best in human and professional behavior. In many ways these people are the unsung heroes and heroines in our fight against AIDS." [109]

THE GLOBAL PICTURE

S ince the first edition of this dossier was published in November 1986, information on the extent of AIDS and HIV infection worldwide has increased. By 30 June 1988 138 out of 176 countries and territories reporting to the World Health Organization (WHO) had cases of AIDS, compared to 102 out of 135 in December 1986. The total number of cases recorded by WHO on that date was 100,410, which represented a doubling time of a little over a year. As discussed in Chapter Three, however, 50% or more of cases may not be reported, especially by countries where lack of financial resources means that surveillance systems are weak.

To gain a more realistic picture of the spread of Aids at a national level, case reports must be related to population size. Calculating the number of cases per million population gives an indication of the relative seriousness of the epidemic between countries with different sizes of populations. On that basis, the following are the 10 leading AIDS-affected countries on officially reported figures.

COUNTRIES MOST AFFECTED BY AIDS

	Officially reported AIDS cases	Population (in millions)	AIDS cases per million population
French Guiana	113	0.082	1,378
Bermuda	75	0.056	1,339
Bahamas	188	0.235	800
Congo	1,250	2.100	595
USA	65,780	243.800	270
Guadeloupe	74	0.300	247
Burundi	1,156	5.000	231
Haiti	1,374	6.200	222
Barbados	55	0.300	183
Trinidad	227	1.300	175

Source: Panos, based on WHO or Ministry of Health figures reported by June 1988, and excluding countries reporting fewer than 10 cases.

In the following pages we give a country by country breakdown of the June 1988 state of the AIDS pandemic. Although the information is not complete, it is, however, the most comprehensive global picture of the situation to date. It includes seroprevalence studies, which give a better guide to the extent of infection, although surveys of specific segments of a population (eg: prostitutes or blood donors in a large city) should not be taken as representative of the country as a whole. Similarly, small samples are less likely to be statistically representative than larger ones.

To save space, information has been compressed and should be interpreted with care. Further details will be available from the references quoted and from the

Ministry of Health or National AIDS Committee in each country. References to press articles are given where few other sources of information for a particular country were available, but readers are cautioned that all statistical data in press articles should be carefully checked for accuracy against primary sources. Headings are explained below:

Cases reported: refers to the number of AIDS cases meeting the US Centers for Disease Control or WHO case definitions of AIDS.

Breakdown: where given, refers to the risk behaviour which is believed to have been the means of transmission of the virus. Thus "10% homosexual contact" means that 10% of people diagnosed with AIDS are believed to have been infected through homosexual activity. The term *ivdu* means intravenous drug user.

Seropositivity: "3/283 (1.1%) hospital patients." This means that 3 out of 283 hospital patients tested, a figure equivalent to 1.1% of the sample, tested positive for HIV antibodies. There is no indication as to how they became infected. "Total of 300,000" means that at the given date in the whole country 300,000 people were estimated to be carrying HIV. "5% in capital" means that 5% of the sexually active adult population (not of the whole population) of the capital is believed to be infected. Unless otherwise stated, seropositive, HIV-positive and HIV+ all refer to HIV-1 (see Chapter One). Where possible date, place and size of sample has been given; otherwise "To [a date]" refers to date of publication.

Action: References to assessment visits, short-term plans (STP), medium-term plans (MTP) and technical services agreements (TSA) are to the status of national AIDS programmes and plans, as developed with the assistance of WHO, at 10 March 1988. A short-term plan is the initial stage of activity and lasts 6 — 12 months; it involves, among other aspects, a review of local knowledge of HIV infection, identification of groups at risk and initial public information and education activities. A medium-term plan lasts 3 to 5 years; among its targets are the linkage of AIDS prevention and control with primary health care strategy, implementation of blood screening and encouraging specific behaviour changes. (For further details see the WHO publication *Guidelines for the development of a national AIDS prevention and control programme*, WHO AIDS Series 1, 1988.)

Entry Restrictions: Where categories are given, eg: "residence applicants", this means that foreign visitors in this category are required to provide certificates showing negative HIV-antibody status. "Foreign students" refers to overseas nationals studying in the country concerned and not to students visiting on holiday.

Abbreviations in the data refer to the following sources:

AACIA : (Abstracts from) the Second International Symposium on AIDS and Associated Cancers in Africa, Naples, October 1987

BMJ : *British Medical Journal*

CP Communication with Panos from Ministry of Health / National AIDS Committee

GDSR : Global Diseases Surveillance Report (published by the Global Epidemiology Working Group, Fort Detrick, Maryland 21701, USA)

GIA : (Abstracts from) the Global Impact of AIDS Conference, London, March 1988

HMC: Presentation at the Health Ministers Conference, London, January 1988

IHT : *International Herald Tribune*

NS   *New Scientist*
PAHO: Pan American Health Organization
PICA: (Abstracts from) the Paris International Conference on AIDS, June 1986
SICA I: Volume I of the Abstracts from the Stockholm International Conference on AIDS, June 1988
SICA II :   Volume II of the Abstracts from the Stockholm International Conference on AIDS, June 1988
WICA :   (Abstracts from) the Washington International Conference on AIDS, June 1987

....

NORTH AMERICA

CANADA
First reported case: 1981 (1979 in retrospect)
Cases reported April 1988: 1,775 (69 per million)
Breakdown: 79.9% homosexual contact, 7.8% heterosexual contact, 4.4% recipient of blood products, 2.6% homosexual and ivdu, 2.1% paediatric, 0.5% ivdu, 2.7% undetermined.
Seropositivity: Total of 50,000 to 75,000 people (0.19% to 0.29% of the population) estimated HIV+ [Federal Centre for AIDS, Health & Welfare Canada]. Ontario and Quebec provinces have highest number of cases of AIDS and HIV, although British Columbia ranks highest on a per capita basis [GDSR, October 1987 and December 1987].

To date the Canadian response to AIDS — both public and governmental — has been muted. Yet, in per capita terms, Canada's AIDS epidemic ranks among the more serious in the world. Of the 21 countries with the largest number of reported cases per capita, 18 are developing countries in Africa, or the Caribbean and Latin America and two are rich countries — the United States and Canada. AIDS cases per capita in Canada exceed those in every European country, several of which have conducted vigorous national information campaigns. Canadian complacency about AIDS is misplaced, say many of the country's public health professionals. "All we have to do is to look at what has happened in the United States, which itself responded very late to its epidemic. We are in danger of repeating their mistake and there is no excuse," says Michael Phair, president of the Canadian AIDS Society.

The Canadian Government has recently extended funding for the Federal Centre for AIDS (FCA), with the centre's original C$39 million budget for 1986 to 1991 supplemented by C$129 through 1993. Funds are distributed as follows: C$48 million for education; C$35 million for research; C$20 million for community innovations and local initiatives; C$10 million for health and social service support including professional education; C$6 million for international activities including the Fifth International Conference on AIDS to be held in Montreal in 1989; and C$10 million for operating budget including laboratories.

Research funding will concentrate on drug trials, vaccine development and seroprevalence studies. Development of a national integrated treatment and support program for people with AIDS that will be community based is a current priority for the centre.

The Canadian Public Health Association (CPHA) receives funding (C$3.17 million over 5 years, 1986-91) from the federal government for education programs complementing those of the FCA. CPHA's current nationwide program was tested for both English and French speaking audiences, with the theme "New Facts for Life" in English and "Pour L'Amour de la Vie" in French. While no nationwide study has been conducted to measure the campaign's effectiveness, a study of knowledge and attitudes on AIDS conducted by the Alberta provincial government showed that while most of the over 1,000 adults polled could identify principal routes of HIV transmission, over 40% still incorrectly believe that AIDS also can be transmitted via mosquito bites or casual contact.

Information on the social, economic and ethnic background of persons with AIDS is not currently available.

Thirty-one community-based groups in Canada have joined loosely to form the Canadian AIDS Society based in Edmonton. Phair argues that the FCA priority activity ought to be AIDS information and education instead of palliative care, especially since health care is in any case a provincial rather than a federal government responsibility. AIDS information campaigns in Canada have so far been carried out by federal and some provincial authorities, but, says Phair, they have mostly been "too tepid, too unfocused and probably ineffective." According to CPHA director David Walters, "response to AIDS in Canada is two or three years behind that of the United States. We have a chance to learn from their experience, but we will lose the opportunity if we don't move faster."

Those charged with AIDS education in Canada worry that vulnerable groups, including native Canadians (Canadian Indians, Métis and Inuit) and young Canadians (aged 12 to 20 years) are not being reached with information on how to avoid HIV. According to one survey [A. King et al, SICA I, p493] of 50,000 young people ranging from 12 to 19 years of age there is a general distrust among Canadian youth of government information. Young people reported a high level of embarrassment about buying condoms.

UNITED STATES

First reported case: 1981 (1969 in retrospect)
Cases reported June 1988: 65,780 (270 per million)
Breakdown: (see below) 62.4% homosexual contact, 18.1% ivdu, 7.3% homosexual/ivdu, 4.1% heterosexual contact, 3.7% blood product recipients, 1.2% children of parent at risk, 3.2% undetermined, 91.5% male, 8.5% female.
Seropositivity: Total of 945,000-1.4 million (0.4-0.6% of population) estimated HIV+ in February 1988 [US Centers for Disease Control]. 5,890/3.9 million (0.15%) servicemen and women and military volunteers [*Washington Post*, 11 February 1988]. 148/9047 (1.6%) pregnant mothers in New York City in December 1987 [*New York Times*, 13 January 1988 reporting unpublished seroprevalence study by the NYC AIDS Surveillance Unit]. 5% of STD clinic outpatients in Baltimore in spring 1987 [*Washington Post*, 2 February 1988]. (For a detailed breakdown of seropositivity rates in different groups see *Morbidity and Mortality Weekly Report*, 18 December 1987, Supplement, CDC.) HIV-2 infection detected in New Jersey in December 1987 [*Morbidity and Mortality Weekly Report*, 29 January 1988, pp33-35].

A total of 450,000 AIDS cases (0.2% of the population) are projected for 1993 by the US Public Health Service.

Entry restrictions: applicants for immigration

Internal regulations: a number of states have proposed or passed laws relating to AIDS.

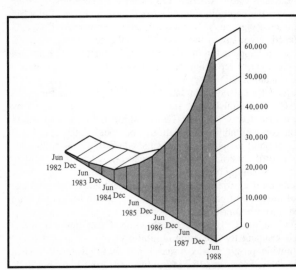

Development of AIDS cases in the USA. (Source: CDC)

Although AIDS was first reported in the USA — and globally — in June 1981, retrospective diagnosis has revealed a number of cases in the late 1970s. The earliest date for which a blood test and symptoms of AIDS in the United States has been confirmed is 1969, in a teenage boy who died that year. The United States currently accounts for 65% of all globally reported cases, a percentage that has been steadily dropping since AIDS first appeared. Current doubling time for cases in the United States is just under 15 months (April 1987 to June 1988).

The above breakdown by risk behaviour refers to all AIDS cases since 1981. Analysis of new cases shows a slowing in the rate of reported cases among homosexual men with no history of drug use. In the last quarter of 1985 they accounted for 68% of new adult cases, while in the second quarter of 1988 they accounted for 56%. In the same period the percentage of cases reported in men and women with a history of drug use has risen from 22% to 32%. The proportion of new cases of women with AIDS has meanwhile risen from 6.4% to over 11%.

A revision of official statistics in New York City in 1987 suggested that ivdus accounted for 53% of all AIDS-related deaths in the city and not 31% as calculated earlier. An estimated 2,520 AIDS-related deaths had not been included in surveillance statistics [*New York Times*, 22 October 1987].

The percentage of people with AIDS who are black or Latino (respectively 26% and 14%) is double that of blacks and Latino in the general population (12% and 7%). The rate has begun to rise steeply in both minority populations, who accounted for over 46% of new cases in the second quarter of 1988. The underlying factors of poverty, drug use and racial discrimination which have led to this overrepresentation of minorities in AIDS case reports in the United States are examined in the Panos book *Blaming Others: Prejudice, race and worldwide AIDS*.

Federal government response to AIDS has been criticised from various quarters, including the Presidential Commission on AIDS, for being too slow and ineffective. The report of the chairman of the Presidential Commission, published in June 1988, made several proposals contrary to current government policy, including calls for federal legal protection against discrimination on grounds of AIDS or HIV infection and wider programmes to prevent spread of the virus amongst drug users. Although federal spending on AIDS-related research and health care has risen steadily fromUS$5.6 million allocated in 1982-83 to almost US$1.3 billion budgeted for 1988-89, the US National Academy of Sciences in its June 1988 report called for further US$3 billion a year by 1990.

The burden of education and health care fell initially on voluntary organisations and later on city and state governments. A wide-ranging series of programmes has sprung up, from the "buddy" system pioneered by Gay Men's Health Crisis in New York City (home care provided by volunteers for people with AIDS) to the bleach and condoms handed out to prostitutes and drug addicts on the streets of San Francisco. As HIV has spread, many of these community-based programmes have become models for prevention and education activities in other countries.

■■■

CARIBBEAN

With populations and economies generally too small to maintain fully independent health services, the English-speaking islands of the Caribbean (with the exception of the US Virgin Islands) all belong to the Caribbean Epidemiology Centre (CAREC) an organisation which was set up in 1975. Three countries on the mainland — Belize, Guyana and Suriname — are also members.

The first cases reported to CAREC were in 1983 from Trinidad. By the end of 1987, 652 cases of AIDS had been reported to CAREC, representing a case rate of 102 per million in an overall population of 6,500,000. Of the 19 member countries

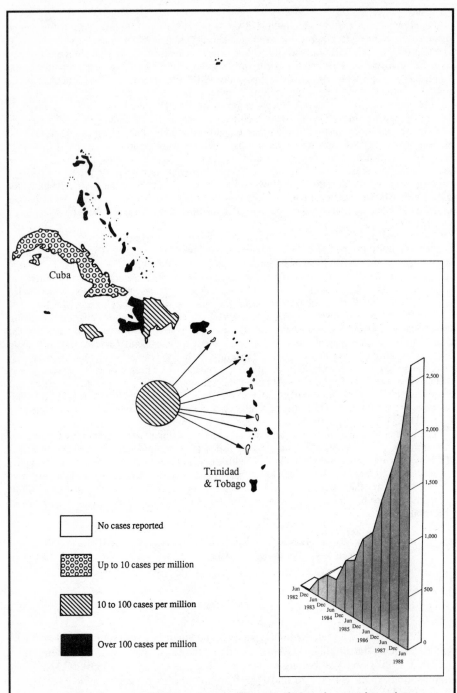

In terms of officially reported AIDS cases per million population, the map shows that some Caribbean countries have the world's most severe AIDS epidemics. The diagram shows cases have been rising steeply since 1984. Source: Panos, from WHO and national health ministry figures up to June 1988.

only two, the British Virgin Islands and Montserrat, reported no cases, while five countries (Bermuda, Bahamas, Barbados, Jamaica, and Trinidad and Tobago) accounted for 90% of the total. The emerging pattern is of an increasingly young and heterosexual population developing AIDS. In the second quarter of 1986, the male:female ratio of new cases was 6:1; a year later it was 2.6:1. In the same period of 1987 the percentage of cases in the 15-29 age group rose from 30% to 52%. Meanwhile a survey of blood donors from eight countries in the latter half of 1986 reported 83 of 8,371 (1%) seropositive. There has been a 150% rise in reported cases of syphilis between 1985 and 1987, with increased reporting only partly attributable to the use of public rather than private medical care. [J. Hospedales, GIA]

CAREC provides laboratory services support, including kits for serological surveys and bulk purchase of items such as gloves. It produces educational material and supplies AIDS counsellors on a short-term basis to train counsellors in member countries. It also screens blood for those countries which do not have their own testing equipment. CAREC also acts as co-ordinator for implementation of WHO national plans. Short term plans have been drawn up for 1988 and medium term plans covering 1989 to 1991 are due to be presented by mid-1988. Blood is already screened in 15 member countries and the remaining four are in the process of acquiring the necessary equipment.

In the French overseas départements of Martinique, Guadeloupe and, on the mainland, French Guiana, AIDS has followed the pattern of rapidly-spreading heterosexual transmission. Early cases in Haiti, the Dominican Republic and Puerto Rico were in homosexual men, probably reflecting the fact that these islands were favourite holiday destinations for gay men from the United States, but in the last two years heterosexual activity has become the predominant means of transmission. Cases of AIDS in the Netherlands Antilles have emerged too recently to suggest a pattern of spread, while no information on risk behaviour has emerged from Cuba.

REPORTED AIDS CASES at June 1988

	Officially reported AIDS cases	Population (in millions)	AIDS cases per million population
Bermuda	75	0.056	1,339
Bahamas	188	0.235	800
Guadeloupe	74	0.300	247
Haiti	1,374	6.200	222
Barbados	55	0.300	183
Trinidad	227	1.300	175
Martinique	38	0.300	127
St Lucia	10	0.100	100
Netherlands Antilles	18	0.200	90
Dominican Republic	504	6.500	78
Jamaica	56	2.500	22
Cuba	27	10.300	3

These figures exclude countries reporting fewer than ten cases. Source: Panos, from WHO and health ministry figures.

Reminder: Seropositivity studies of a specific segment of a population (eg prostitutes or blood donors in a large city) should *not* be taken as representative of the country as a whole.

ANGUILLA (member of CAREC)
No AIDS cases reported or seroprevalence studies published by June 1988. An education campaign began in the summer of 1987.

ANTIGUA (member of CAREC)
First reported case: 1985
Cases reported June 1987: 3 (30 per million)
Action: Assessment visit made.

BAHAMAS (member of CAREC)
First reported case: 1985 (post-diagnosed cases in 1981/2)
Cases reported March 1988: 188 (800 per million)
Action: Assessment visit made.

Fifty per cent of AIDS cases are in Haitians; the pattern of transmission is heterosexual. No ivdu case reported. Overall the rate of venereal disease is very high. There is an AIDS-dedicated ward in the Princess Margaret Hospital [*The Voice*, London, 12 January 1988].

BARBADOS (member of CAREC)
First reported case: 1984
Cases reported December 1987: 55 (183 per million)
Breakdown: 83.6% male, 16.4% female. 40.0% homosexual contact, 7.2% paediatric, 3.6% blood product recipients.
Seropositivity: To June 1987: 1/1,439 (0.07%) blood donors [PAHO, 9 November 1988].
Action: Assessment visit made.

Intravenous drug use has not been a factor in any case of AIDS. A national education campaign began in 1985.

BERMUDA (member of CAREC)
First reported case: 1984
Cases reported September 1987: 75 (1,339 per million)
Breakdown: 62% ivdu.
Seropositivity: To June 1987: 0/508 blood donors [PAHO, 9 November 1987].
Action: Assessment visit made.

BRITISH VIRGIN ISLANDS (member of CAREC)
No cases reported by June 1988.
Seropositivity: 0/50 blood donors.
Action: Assessment visit made. An AIDS education programme began in 1985.

CAYMAN ISLANDS (member of CAREC)
First reported case: 1986
Cases reported December 1987: 3 (150 per million).
Action: Assessment visit made.

CUBA
First reported case: 1986
Cases reported January 1988: 27 (3 per million)
Seropositivity: To January 1988: 174/1,534,993 (0.01%), tests include all blood donations,

pregnant women, hospital admissions, prisoners on entry and release, patients with STDs, haemophiliacs and Cuban personnel working abroad [HMC].
Action: MTP agreed.
Entry restrictions: foreigners staying longer than 3 months.
Internal regulations: quarantine for all individuals with HIV or AIDS.

Cuban exiles in the United States claim seroprevalence in Cuba is much higher than acknowledged in official government statistics [*New York Times*, 11 February 1988]. The government is screening all citizens for HIV. Those found seropositive are interned in a sanatorium in the suburbs of Havana, where they "work, receive visits, are paid 100% of their wages, practise gymnastics, sports, visit tourist places and their relatives are cared for in all aspects by social workers who help them solve any difficulty" [HMC]. Occasional home visits also apparently allowed [*Washington Post*, 16 September 1987; *Miami Herald*, 17 September 1987]. US$5 million has been budgeted on AIDS prevention, treatment and research. Transfusion blood screened since 1986.

DOMINICA (member of CAREC)
First reported case: December 1986
Cases reported June 1987: 6 (60 per million)
Breakdown: 1 child, 1 woman, 4 homosexual men.
Seropositivity: In 1987: 9/92 (10%) of individuals at high risk [HMC].
Action: STP from autumn 1988.

Seropositive cases include 7 homosexual men, some of whom have also had sex with women. A seropositive man passed the virus to his wife, the island's only female case, who passed it on to their child. Both the woman and child have died [HMC]. An AIDS education campaign covering schools, medical personnel, farm-workers and other groups began in January 1987.

DOMINICAN REPUBLIC
First reported case: 1982
Cases reported December 1987: 504 (78 per million)
Breakdown: In 1983 no women had been diagnosed with AIDS; by 1987 32% of all cases were women; 43% of new cases in 1987 were the result of heterosexual transmission [E. Guerrero et al, SICA II, p239].
Seropositivity: In 1986: 14/959 (1.5%) blood donors, 10/521 (1.9%), 12/986 (1.2%) prostitutes [PAHO, 9 November 1987]; in homosexual men, 4.9% in 1983, 18.8% in 1984, 12.9% in 1985.
Action: STP completed.

According to the director of the country's STD study programme, the spread of AIDS to heterosexuals has been speeded by high levels of prostitution, venereal disease and the return of infected nationals from the United States [*Miami Herald*, 15 September 1987]. Condom use reportedly has risen dramatically in the Dominican Republic, reaching 71% of males and 48% of female sex workers by October 1987 [A. A. de Moya & E Guerrero, SICA II, p275].

GRENADA (member of CAREC)
First reported case: 1984 (post mortem diagnosis)
Cases reported January 1988: 8 (80 per million population)
Action: AIDS Prevention Task Force set up in 1986; MTP from May 1988.

Five people reported seropositive. According to the Minister of Health several factors make Grenada particularly vulnerable to AIDS — tourism, drug-trafficking, seasonal farm-workers in the United States and the periodic return of thousands of Grenadians living abroad [HMC].

GUADELOUPE (Overseas Département of France)
First reported case: 1982

Cases reported December 1987: 74 (247 per million population)
Seropositivity: In 1986: 16/9,356 (0.2%) blood donors [PAHO, 9 November 1987].

Homosexual contact is the means of transmission in only 7% of AIDS cases in the French Départements of the Caribbean (Guadeloupe, Martinique and French Guiana). Drug addiction is responsible for 1%. Children account for 10% of all cases, while in mid-1986 42% of those who were ill were women [*Le Monde*, Paris, 14 October 1987].

HAITI
First reported case: 1983
Cases reported September 1987: 1,374 (222 per million)
Breakdown at 3rd quarter 1987: 51% urban, 45% rural, 4% provenance unknown; 69.7% male, 30.3% female; 56.4% risk category undetermined, 25.7% heterosexual contact, 10.0% blood product recipients, 2.1% homosexual contact, 5.8% children.
Action: STP completed.

Kaposi's sarcoma as an opportunistic infection has decreased from 19% to 5%. The percentage of cases outside Port-au-Prince, the capital, rose from 11% to 30% between 1983 and 1987. Infection with HIV is associated with high mortality in children even before the onset of AIDS [J. W. Pape et al, GIA, p40].

Until 1985 the US Centers for Disease Control classified Haitians as a risk category equivalent to homosexuals, haemophiliacs and heroin addicts. The effects of this categorisation on Haitians in the United States and on Haiti itself are analysed in the Panos book *Blaming Others: Prejudice, race and worldwide AIDS*. Transfusion blood is screened only in Port-au-Prince.

JAMAICA (member of CAREC)
First reported case: 1983
Cases reported January 1988: 56 (22 per million)
Breakdown: By September 1987: 63.3% men, 26.7% women, 10.0% children.
Seropositivity: In 1987: 13/5,724 (0.2%) blood donors [PAHO], 127/27,000 (0.5%) blood samples [*Daily Gleaner*, 15 September 1987].
Action: MTP from autumn 1988.
Entry restrictions: reported to be under discussion.

Reported AIDS cases rose fourfold between December 1986 and December 1987. The majority of cases reported by September 1987 resulted from heterosexual contact, 23% from homosexual contact [J. P. Figueroa et al, GIA, p40]. An education campaign began in 1986. Blood donations fell sharply when screening began but have now returned to previous levels. In early 1988 a survey of the population's attitudes towards and knowledge of AIDS was begun preparatory to a second phase of the media campaign.

MARTINIQUE (Overseas Département of France)
First reported case: 1983
Cases reported December 1987: 38 (127 per million)
Breakdown: see Guadeloupe
Seropositivity: In 1986: 20/10,109 (0.2%) blood donors [*Bulletin Épidémiologique Hebdomadaire*, 11/1987].

MONTSERRAT (member of CAREC)
No cases of AIDS reported by June 1988.
Seropositivity: Of 88 blood donors tested in 1987, all but one, a "borderline positive" case, were seronegative [CP].

NETHERLANDS ANTILLES
First reported case: 1987
Cases reported June 1987: 18 (90 per million)
Seropositivity: In 1987: 2/1,221 (0.2%) blood donors [PAHO, 9 November 1987].

PUERTO RICO (US Commonwealth)
Cases reported May 1988: 1,006 (291 per million)
(Puerto Rico figures are included in US statistics.)

SAINT CHRISTOPHER AND NEVIS (member of CAREC)
First reported case: 1985
Cases reported September 1987: 1 (22 per million)
Action: Assessment visit made.

SAINT LUCIA (member of CAREC)
First reported case: 1984
Cases reported January 1988: 10 (100 per million)
Breakdown: At October 1987: 1 homosexual man, 4 heterosexual men, 4 women.
Seropositivity: In 1985: 5/560 (0.9%) farmworkers. 1986: 1/340 (0.3%) general population.
Action: Assessment visit made.

Education campaign began in 1985. At particular risk are 500 farmworkers who annually spend seven or eight months in Belle Glade, Florida, where high levels of seropositivity and AIDS have been recorded.

SAINT VINCENT AND GRENADINES (member of CAREC)
First reported case: 1985
Cases reported December 1987: 8 (80 per million)
Action: Assessment visit made.

TRINIDAD AND TOBAGO (member of CAREC)
First reported case: 1983
Cases reported December 1987: 227 (175 per million)
Breakdown: At January 1987: 75% homosexual contact, 12% women, 10% pediatric. At December 1987: 63% homosexual contact, 22% heterosexual contact.
Seropositivity: In 1987: 59/6,407 (0.9%) blood donors [PAHO, 9 November 1987]; 3.3% of 506 STD patients [C. Bartholomew et al, SICA II, p240].
Action: MTP completed.

Initial AIDS cases resulting from heterosexual contact were in women with bisexual partners, but 16 of the 22 heterosexual cases reported in 1987 were in men whose only risk activity was frequent sexual contact with women [F. R. Cleghorn et al, GIA, p55].

TURKS AND CAICOS ISLANDS (member of CAREC)
First reported case: 1986
Cases reported December 1987: 5 (625 per million)
Action: MTP from autumn 1988.

US VIRGIN ISLANDS (US Territory)
Cases reported May 1988: 16 (152 per million)
(US Virgin Islands figures are included in US statistics.)

....

CENTRAL AND SOUTH AMERICA

REPORTED AIDS CASES at June 1988

	Officially reported AIDS cases	Population (in millions)	AIDS cases per million population
French Guiana	113	0.82	1,378
Honduras	149	4.70	32
Brazil	2,956	141.50	21
Guyana	14	0.80	18
Mexico	1,302	81.90	16
Costa Rica	43	2.80	15
Panama	30	2.30	13
Venezuela	140	18.30	8
Uruguay	20	3.10	6
Colombia	174	29.90	6
Chile	69	12.40	6
Argentina	163	31.50	5
El Salvador	25	5.30	5
Guatemala	34	8.40	4
Ecuador	39	10.00	4
Peru	69	20.70	3

The above figures exclude countries reporting fewer than 10 cases. Source: Panos, from PAHO and health ministry figures

AIDS first appeared in the region in homosexual men and recipients of blood products. Although these two groups still form the majority of cases in most countries, there is evidence of increasing heterosexual spread. Countries with a high percentage of cases in women include French Guiana (35%) and Honduras (38%). Although such countries as Bolivia and Colombia are a major source of illegal drugs, injection is not common and is not a principal means of transmission of HIV.

A factor expected to influence the spread of AIDS in Latin America is the high proportion of men who marry but have sexual relations with other men: (see discussion in Chapter Three). An additional factor, particularly in Brazil, is the large number of *travestis* (transvestite men who live as women and take hormones to develop their breasts but without losing their male genitalia) in urban prostitution.

Most countries in the region have relatively high standards of health care in comparison with Africa and much of Asia, though much of it is privately funded. However, existing health services will be placed under increasing pressure as the number of AIDS cases grows. In Central America particularly, there is concern that thousands of individuals will return from the United States having been refused residence in that country because they are seropositive.

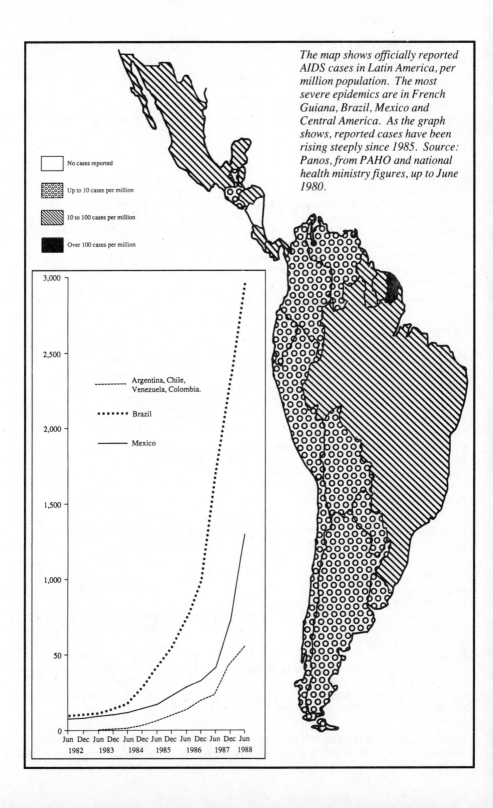

The map shows officially reported AIDS cases in Latin America, per million population. The most severe epidemics are in French Guiana, Brazil, Mexico and Central America. As the graph shows, reported cases have been rising steeply since 1985. Source: Panos, from PAHO and national health ministry figures, up to June 1980.

No cases reported

Up to 10 cases per million

10 to 100 cases per million

Over 100 cases per million

Argentina, Chile, Venezuela, Colombia.

Brazil

Mexico

Three countries in Central and South America, Belize, Guyana and Suriname, are members of CAREC (see Caribbean section) but are listed in this section.

For information on Pan American Health Organization activity in the region, see Chapter Eight.

Reminder: Seropositivity studies of a specific segment of a population (eg prostitutes or blood donors in a large city) should *not* be taken as representative of the country as a whole.

ARGENTINA
First reported case: 1983
Cases reported March 1988: 163 (5 per million)
Breakdown: at April 1986: 92% homosexual, 6% haemophiliac; 100% male.
Seropositivity: January to December 1987: 11/28,176 (0.04%) blood donors, the majority from Buenos Aires, Rosario and Tucumán provinces [O Fay et al, SICA I, p347]. To June 1988: 646/2528 (26%) individuals at high risk [G. Muchinik et al, SICA I, p330], reaching 60% of 101 ivdus [P. Cahn et al, SICA I, p331]; 64/376 (17%) male and female prisoners (all but two seropositives heterosexual ivdus) [J. Benetucci et al, SICA I, p312].
Action: MTP completed.

Transfusion blood was not screened at the end of 1987.

BELIZE (member of CAREC)
First reported case: 1986
Cases reported December 1987: 7 (35 per million)
Action: STP completed March 1988.
Entry restrictions: applicants for residence, work permits and naturalisation.

BOLIVIA
First reported case: October 1985
Cases reported January 1988: 6 (0.9 per million).
Breakdown: All homosexual men, 1 Canadian, 5 Bolivian.
Seropositivity: To November 1987, Santa Cruz region: 0/333 female prostitutes, 0/12 homosexual men [F. Paradisi et al, SICA I, p334].
Action: Assessment visit completed.

The first three AIDS cases are believed to have contracted AIDS abroad (in Brazil, Canada and the United States). The next three cases are all prisoners who are believed to have contracted the virus in La Paz. Transfusion blood was not screened at the end of 1987.

BRAZIL
First reported case: 1982
Cases reported April 1988: 2,956 (21 per million)
Breakdown: at December 1987: 71.0% homosexual contact, 9.0% blood product recipient, 6.4% ivdu, 5.6% heterosexual contact; 56.9% in São Paulo state, 19.1% in Rio de Janeiro state; 94.5% male, 5.5% female.
Seropositivity: To June 1988: 52/284 (18.3%) women prisoners in Sao Paulo, ivdu drug use major risk factor [Q. W. Rodriguez et al, SICA I, p313]; 5/70 (7.1%) "professional" blood donors [M. I. Carvalho et al, SICA, p347]; 31/132 (24%) homosexual men (HIV-1+) [E. Cortes, SICA I, p331]. HIV-2 detected in 1/177 (0.6%) female prostitutes, 4/132 (3%) homosexual men, 3/140 (2.1%) AIDS patients [as previous reference].
Action: MTP completed.

Although notification of AIDS is mandatory many cases are unreported, particularly among the middle-class, who have access to private doctors and hospitals. ["O Impacto Social Da AIDS No Brasil", ABIA, Rio de Janeiro, January 1988]. The true total of AIDS cases is believed to be up to 50% higher. Figures from Rio de Janeiro suggest 17.9% of cases there are caused by contaminated blood and 1.3% of cases attributable to drug use or contaminated needles. Approximately 5,500,000 units of blood are transfused each year in Brazil and the government has announced its intention to ensure that it is all screened by June 1988.

Several factors make Brazil particularly vulnerable to AIDS. It has an exceptionally young and sexually active population (50% are under 21 and 70% under 30). Thirty-three per cent of all pregnancies and 26% of all abortions are in teenagers [HMC]. Condoms have not been in common use, although there has been an upsurge in demand in the last year. Many men are bisexual (see introduction to this section) and in the large cities there are many bars, cinemas and public saunas where indiscriminate homosexual activity takes place.

The government has acknowledged the role played by voluntary organisations and invited a founding member of at least one, the Grupo Gay de Bahia, onto the national AIDS committee.

CHILE
First reported case: 1984
Cases reported March 1988: 69 (6 per million)
Breakdown: at September 1987: 75% homosexual contact, 12% heterosexual contact, 5% ivdu.
Seropositivity: reported to be 0.008% of blood donors [GDSR January 1988].
Action: STP completed.

Transfusion blood is screened.

COLOMBIA
First reported case: 1984
Cases reported December 1987: 174 (6 per million) 97% homo/bisexual men; 84% 20-39 years old.
Seropositivity: Of 3,000 homosexual men tested at an unknown date 16% were seropositive [CP]. To June 1988: 14% homosexual men in Bogotá, 4% homosexual men in Villavicencio (sample sizes unknown) HIV+; 0.009% of 38,077 blood donors in 7 cities; 1/762 Amerindian (0.1%) [J. Boshell et al, SICA I, p334].
Action: Assessment visit completed.

COSTA RICA
First reported case: 1983
Cases reported January 1988: 43 (15 per million)
Breakdown: 30% haemophiliac.
Seropositivity: In 1987: 21/18,770 (0.1%) blood donors, 41/58 (70%) and 58/105 (55%) haemophiliacs, 10-20% homosexual men [PAHO].
Action: Assessment visit completed.
Entry restrictions: Foreign students and applicants for residence. An earlier restriction on foreign seamen has been repealed.

250 new cases predicted in 1992, giving total of 690 cases [L. Mata et al, SICA II, p239]. Transfusion blood screened in Red Cross and Social Security blood banks since 1985 and in some private blood banks.

ECUADOR
First reported case: 1985
Cases reported March 1988: 39 (4 per million)
Breakdown: At January 1988: 43.3% homosexual men, 40.0% bisexual men, 6.7% heterosexual (sex unstated), 10.0% blood transfusion.
Action: MTP completed.

At the end of 1987 transfusion blood screened in Red Cross blood banks in Quito and Guayaquil.

EL SALVADOR
First reported case: 1985
Cases reported January 1988: 25 (5 per million)
Action: STP completed.

At the end of 1987 transfusion blood screened only in Red Cross blood bank in San Salvador.

FALKLAND ISLANDS (Malvinas)
No AIDS cases reported or seroprevalence studies published by June 1988. An announcement that blood tests on the entire population (2,000) to be carried out in 1988 would include the HIV-antibody test [*Times*, London, 23 April 1988] has not been confirmed [*Guardian*, London, 21 June 1988].

FRENCH GUIANA (Département of France)
First reported case: 1983
Cases reported March 1988: 113 (1,378 per million)
Breakdown: at March 1987: 51% heterosexual men, 35% heterosexual women, 12% children of parents at risk, 1% homosexual/ivdu, 1% blood product recipient.
Seropositivity: In 1986: 8/2,846 (0.3%) blood donors [PAHO].

The first 32 cases of AIDS were all reported to be in immigrants, the majority from Haiti. An education campaign began in July 1987 in co-ordination with the French Caribbean Départements of Guadeloupe and Martinique.

GUATEMALA
First reported case: 1985
Cases reported December 1987: 34 (4 per million)
Breakdown: 29 men, 3 women, 2 unstated; 25 homosexual contact, 2 ivdu, 1 blood product recipient, rest unstated; 70% had lived in the USA, 10% non-Guatemalan.
Seropositivity: December 1987: total of 26 HIV+ identified.
Action: Assessment visit planned.

At the end of 1987 transfused blood was not screened.

GUYANA (member of CAREC)
First reported case: 1987
Cases reported December 1987: 14 (18 per million)
Action: MTP from autumn/winter 1988.

Unconfirmed report in November 1987 suggested first 12 cases of AIDS were in homosexual men who had travelled frequently.

HONDURAS
First reported case: 1985
Cases reported June 1988: 149 (32 per million)
Breakdown: 63.8% heterosexual contact, 19.7% homosexual contact, 10.7% bisexual, 2.0% children of infected mothers, 1.3% blood product recipients, 0.7% ivdu, 2.0% unknown 38% women.
Seropositivity: In June 1988: total of 74 seropositive, in addition to 65 with blood samples waiting to be confirmed and 7 with AIDS-related complex.
Action: Assessment visit completed.

Of the 95 cases resulting from heterosexual transmission, 14 were prostitute women. Transfusion blood in major hospitals has been screened since August 1987; remaining hospitals are being equipped.

MEXICO
First reported case: 1981
Cases reported April 1988: 1,302 (16 per million)
Breakdown: At October 1987: 87.2% homosexual contact, 7.8% blood products, 4.2% heterosexual contact, 0.5% perinatal, 0.3% ivdu; 95.5% male, 4.5% female; 42.7% of cases in the capital (Federal District).
Seropositivity: To April 1987: 0.4% of unpaid blood donors, 5.5% of paid donors to blood banks [*Boletín Mensual* SIDA, Ano 1, no 2, 15 April 1987]. Dec 1986-Dec 1987: 3/670 (0.4%) female prostitutes in Guadalajara [B. M. Torres-Mendoza, SICA I, p332]. Aug 1985-Dec1987: 119/389 (30.6%) homosexual men in Guadalajara [E. Vázquez-Valls et al, SICA I, p332].
Action: MTP planned.

By 1991 heterosexual transmission predicted to be responsible for 12.6% of cases and blood product recipients for 14-18% of cases [J. Sepúlveda et al, SICA I, p 346; M. A. Lezana et al, SICA II, p233]. Transfusion blood has been screened since September 1987.

NICARAGUA
Cases reported: No cases of AIDS reported to WHO (see below).
Action: Assessment visit planned.

Earlier reports of 19 AIDS cases were withdrawn in May 1988. It was reported in late 1987 that the government was planning a US$1 million AIDS education campaign. Transfusion blood was not screened at the end of 1987. The national AIDS campaign has been drawn up in collaboration with the Nicaragua AIDS Education Project, a San Francisco-based group of health workers [D. Wohlfeiler, SICA II, p 270].

PANAMA
First reported case: 1984
Cases reported December 1987: 30 (13 per million) 30% haemophiliac.
Seropositivity: In 1986: 4/6279 (0.1%) [PAHO]. August 1987: 0.47% of 17,001 military personnel [M. Pereira et al, SICA I, p336].
Action: Assessment visit completed.

A report in late 1987 suggested there had been 30 AIDS deaths and 112 individuals identified as seropositive [GDSR. Dec 1987]. Transfusion blood screened in 10 regions, covering 97% of the country.

PARAGUAY
First reported case: 1986
Cases reported December 1987: 8 (2 per million)
Action: Assessment visit completed.

PERU
First reported case: 1983
Cases reported December 1987: 69 (3 per million)
Seropositivity: 1987: 9/124 (7.3%) haemophiliacs [PAHO]; 1% of 16,000 people at risk [El Comercio, Lima, 15 September 1987]. December 1987: 192/33,623 (0.6%) samples [G. Aguero & M. Lujan, SICA I, p333]. To June 1988: 175/35,526 (0.5%) samples, with highest rate of 83/1,236 (6.7%) in homosexual men [G. Aguero et al, SICA I, p334.]
Action: National Multisectoral Program for the Prevention of AIDS set up in April 1987; assessment visit completed.

Other sources [G. Aguero & M. Lujan above and E. Gotuzzo, SICA I, p334], give 100+ and 88 AIDS cases respectively. Transfusion blood was not screened in December 1987.

SURINAME (member of CAREC)
First reported case: 1984
Cases reported December 1987: 9 (23 per million).
Seropositivity: April - June 1987: 1/236 (0.4%) blood donors.
Action: STP completed March 1988.

URUGUAY
First reported case: 1983
Cases reported March 1988: 20 (6 per million)
Breakdown: At December 1987: 100% homo/bisexual men.
Seropositivity: To September 1987: 102/214 (47.7%) homosexual men, 3/36 (8.3%) haemophiliacs, 3/342 (0.9%) prostitutes, 0/591 blood donors [CP].
Action: Assessment visit completed.

An education campaign began in August 1987.

VENEZUELA
First reported case: 1983
Cases reported December 1987: 140 (8 per million)
Breakdown: Of first 95 cases: 76.8% homo-/bisexual men, 8.4% blood product recipients, 7.4% heterosexual men, 4.2% heterosexual women, 1.1% ivdu, 2.1% unknown; 93.6% male, 6.4% female.
Seropositivity: To November 1987: 1/1,508 (0.1%) blood donors, 84/407 (20.6%) homo-/bisexual men [PAHO].
Action: National Commission for the Study of AIDS set up in mid-1984, now integrated into a National AIDS Commission.

The first AIDS cases were in middle/upper class homo/bisexual men who contracted HIV abroad. Cases are now seen in poorer classes and as the result of infection in Venezuela. The majority of early heterosexual cases were in men and women from Haiti. Transfusion blood screened since 1986.

■■■-

EUROPE

In Western Europe cases of AIDS have followed Pattern I (see Chapter Three) with a striking shift towards intravenous drug users in many countries including Italy, Spain and Yugoslavia. In Eastern Europe seropositivity was first detected in 1985 and cases of AIDS appeared the following year. With the exception of Yugoslavia, infection was originally restricted to haemophiliacs and homosexual men but has recently begun to appear in women. Several Eastern European countries, notably Bulgaria, Czechoslovakia and the Soviet Union, accept large numbers of students from the Third World; an estimated 350 from Africa have tested seropositive and been deported.

Shortages of condoms are reported in almost every Eastern European country, and those condoms which are available are often substandard. Reuse of unsterilised needles/syringes is common due to shortages, and in the Soviet Union it is feared that HIV could be spread by this means, as epidemics of Hepatitis A have been. Homosexuality, intravenous drug use and alcoholism (leading to unprotected sex) are probable risk activities in a number of East European countries. Donated blood has been increasingly screened.

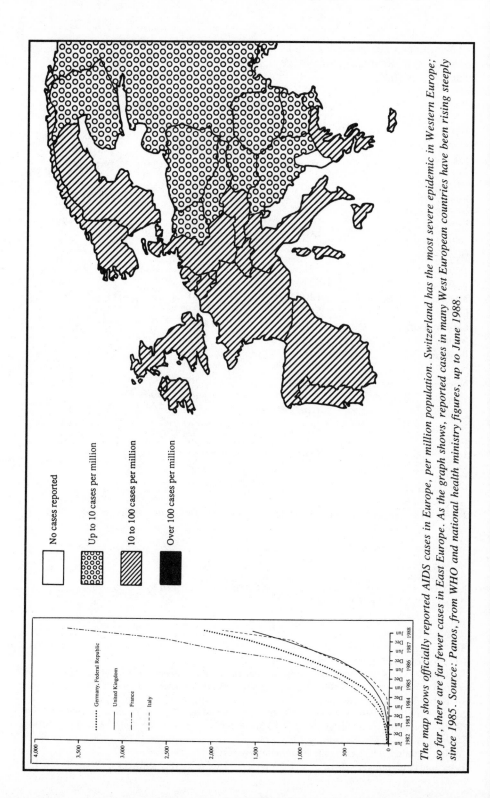

The map shows officially reported AIDS cases in Europe, per million population. Switzerland has the most severe epidemic in Western Europe; so far, there are far fewer cases in East Europe. As the graph shows, reported cases in many West European countries have been rising steeply since 1985. Source: Panos, from WHO and national health ministry figures, up to June 1988.

Reminder: Seropositivity studies of a specific segment of a population (eg prostitutes or blood donors in a large city) should not be taken as representative of the country as a whole.

REPORTED AIDS CASES at June 1988

	Officially reported AIDS cases	Population (in millions)	AIDS cases per million population
Switzerland	439	6.60	67
France	3,628	55.60	65
Denmark	263	5.10	52
Netherlands	526	14.60	36
Belgium	340	9.90	34
West Germany	2,091	61.00	34
Italy	1,865	57.40	32
Spain	1,126	39.00	29
UK	1,541	56.80	27
Luxembourg	10	.040	25
Malta	10	.040	25
Sweden	197	8.40	23
Austria	176	7.60	23
Norway	81	4.20	19
Portugal	125	10.30	12
Greece	106	10.00	11
Ireland	37	3.50	11
Finland	27	4.90	6
Yugoslavia	38	23.40	2
Hungary	12	10.60	1
Czechoslovakia	10	15.60	.6

These figures exclude countries reporting fewer than 10 cases. Source: Panos, from WHO and health ministry figures.

ALBANIA
No AIDS cases reported or seroepidemiological surveys published by March 1988.
Action: STP, TSA from October 1987.

AUSTRIA
First reported case: 1983
Cases reported May 1988: 176 (23 per million)
Breakdown: In April 1986: 65% homosexual men. By February 1988: 48.3% homosexual contact, 25.2% ivdu, 11.9% blood product recipients, 10.6% undetermined, 2.6% heterosexual contact, 1.3% ivdu/homosexual.
Seropositivity: To February 1987: 200/300,000 (0.07%) blood tests. To January 1988: 8/1,300 (0.6%) licensed prostitutes in Vienna (6 were ivdus and the other two partners of ivdus) [*Independent*, London, 11 January 1988].
Action: National AIDS Committee formed in August 1985.
Internal regulations: licensed prostitutes undergo HIV test every six weeks, licence is revoked

if found positive but they are then eligible for state pension of US$450 a month [*Independent*, London, 11 January 1988].

An earlier report that the city of Klagenfurt would refuse work permits to foreigners who could not prove they were HIV-negative was described as "meaningless" by the Austrian Embassy in London.

BELGIUM
First reported case: 1983
Cases reported by May 1988: 340 (34 per million)
Breakdown: at September 1987:63.2% non-residents 36.8% residents

	residents	non-residents
homo/bisexual men	55.9%	5.1%
heterosexual men & women	21.6%	75.4%
recipients of blood products	9.8%	6.3%
ivdu	2.0%	1.1%
homosexual/ivdu	2.0%	0.6%
other risk factors	5.9%	6.9%
undetermined	2.9%	4.6%
men, all risk factors	81.4%	69.7%
women, all risk factors	18.6%	30.3%

Sixty-five per cent of non-residents with AIDS by September 1987 were from Zaire; another 14% come from elsewhere in Africa; the majority of the rest were Belgians who had been living abroad. Seropositivity: To September 1987: confirmed in 2,512 individuals; total believed to be about 10,000 (0.1% of the population. ["SIDA en Belgique, Situation au 30 septembre 1987", Institut d'Hygiène et d'Épidémologie, Brussels].
Entry restrictions: Foreign recipients of certain government scholarships.

BULGARIA
First reported case: 1987
Cases reported October 1987: 3 (0.3 per million)
Seropositivity: To December 1987: 51/260,613 (0.02%) citizens, 51/26,651 (0.81%) non-citizens [GDSR, December 1987]. To June 1988: total of 127 HIV+ detected, of which at least 76 Bulgarian and 31 foreign; 1/500 pregnant women HIV+ [BTA press releases, 21 June 1988 and May 1988].
Action: STP drawn up.
Entry restrictions: Foreigners staying longer than 30 days.
Compulsory testing: pregnant women, citizens returning from working abroad, newly-married couples; "Bulgaria is to test all citizens between 14 and 70 by 1990" [*Financial Times*, London, 6 April 1988].

All non-Bulgarians carrying the virus deported. "Specialised services" for testing for HIV infection were set up at border checkpoints in late December [IHT, 23 December 1987]. Legislation on AIDS is being developed to "protect asymptomatic HIV-carriers from discrimination and to guarantee [their] personal dignity" [HMC].

CZECHOSLOVAKIA
First reported case: 1984
Cases reported March 1988: 10 (0.6 per million)
Breakdown: At December 1987: 6 homosexual contact, 2 undetermined.
Seropositivity: To December 1987: 0/215,382 blood donors, 13/669 (2%) haemophiliacs,

25/1,589 (1.6%) homo/bisexuals [M. Bruckova et al, SICA I, p305]. To June 1988: 59 Czechs and Slovaks HIV+, of which 37 homosexual, 16 haemophiliac, 3 heterosexual men and 3 women infected by their partners; total of 500-1,000 believed HIV+ [CPK press release, 22 June 1988].
Entry restrictions: Foreign students.

Two suspected cases of AIDS pre-1984 died before seropositivity tests available. At least 16 foreigners who tested positive have been deported. Transfusion blood officially screened since January 1987 but reports differ as to the extent of blood screening.

DENMARK
First reported case: 1980 [in retrospect]
Cases reported May 1988: 263   (52 per million)
Breakdown: At July 1987: 96.6% men, 3.4% women. At December 1987: 84% homosexual contact, 5% blood product recipient, 5% heterosexual contact, 2% ivdu, 2% ivdu/homosexual, 3% others/undetermined.
Seropositivity: To January 1988: estimated 10-35% of homosexual men, 15-30% ivdus, 30% of haemophiliacs; 12/600,000 (0.002%) blood donations in 1986 and 1987 (all 12 had known risk factors) [GDSR, January 1988].
Action: National AIDS Secratariat set up in November 1987.

By March 1987 more than 70% of AIDS cases were in the Copenhagen area. The information campaign in Denmark has been among the most imaginative in the world, including AIDS education buses with 3 metre long condoms painted on the side.

FINLAND
First reported case: 1984
Cases reported March 1988: 27 (6 per million)
Breakdown: At August 1987: 90% male, 10% female. At December 1987: 71% homosexual contact, 17% heterosexual contact, 8% blood product recipients.
Seropositivity: To August 1987: 5/350,000 blood donations, 0/5,000 pregnant women, 23/6,300 (0.4%) STD patients, 8/1,500 (0.5%) "anonymously tested people" [CP]. To June 1988: 1/9,738 pregnant women (99.6% of all pregnant women in time period) [M.L. Kantanen et al, SICA II, p219].
Entry restrictions: there are conflicting reports as to whether foreign students are required to undergo testing.

Both AIDS and HIV spreading at a rate substantially lower than other Western European countries. Pamphlet on AIDS sent to every household in June 1986. Campaign budget for 1987 was US$800,000.

FRANCE
First reported case: 1981 (post diagnosis)
Cases reported March 1988: 3,628 (65 per million)
Breakdown: Adult cases up to March 1988: 60.6% homosexual contact, 12.6% ivdu, 10.1% heterosexual contact, 7.7% blood product recipients, 2.9% homosexual/ivdu, 6.0% undetermined; male:female ratio 6.8:1. 101 of the 3,628 (2.8%) cases are in children. New cases in 1988: 53.6% homosexual men, 17.2% ivdus [*Bulletin Épidémiologique Hebdomadaire*, 19/1988, 16 May 1988].
Seropositivity: 0.03% of general population (0.15% in Paris), with total of 150,000-250,000 [National Blood Transfusion Society quoted in *Le Monde*, Paris, 7-8 February 1988]. HIV-2 detected in 9/10,004 (0.09%) individuals at risk and 0/100,114 blood donations; 30/100,114 (0.03%) blood donations HIV-1+ [A. M. Courouce, SICA II, p223]. In prisons between 0.5% and 15% according to region [*Le Monde*, Paris, 9 March 1988].

FFr930 million budgeted for prevention, health care and education in 1988 [*Nature*, 1988, 331

(Jan 14) p106 & (Jan 28) p290]. In 1987 the government education campaign slogan was "Le sida, il ne passera pas par moi" (AIDS won't pass my way). Free and anonymous screening for HIV is being introduced at special centres throughout the country.

GERMAN DEMOCRATIC REPUBLIC (EAST GERMANY)
First reported case: December 1986, haemophiliac
Cases reported December 1987: 6 (0.4 per million)
Breakdown: 2 homosexual, 2 haemophiliac, 2 undetermined.
Seropositivity: To March 1988: 38 citizens, 70 foreigners [ADN, press release, 24 March 1988].
Action: National AIDS Committee set up in 1983.

It was reported in January 1988 that proof of HIV-negativity would be demanded of East Germans travelling to the USSR and of foreigners staying in East Germany "for a long time" [*Neues Deutschland*, quoted in *Le Monde*, Paris, 5 January 1988]. An education campaign began in March 1987. Transfusion blood screened since 1986.

GERMANY, FEDERAL REPUBLIC (WEST GERMANY)
First reported case: 1982
Cases reported May 1988: 2,091 (34 per million)
Breakdown: at December 1987: 75% homosexual contact, 9% ivdu, 7% blood product recipients, 3% heterosexual contact, 1% homosexual contact/ivdu, 5% other/undetermined.
Seropositivity: In 1986: 9/1,800 (0.5%) pregnant women in Berlin (including 7 from high-risk groups) [NS London, 21 January 1987]. HIV-2 detected in February 1987 [K.A.E. Weber, SICA II, p223].
Entry restrictions: Recipients of certain government scholarships; certain visa holders "if they fall ill" (see below).
Internal restrictions: See below

Entry visas issued to students and business travellers from certain African countries are stamped "Erlischt bei gesundheitlichen Bedenken" (May be rendered invalid on health grounds). The Land of Bavaria has obligatory blood tests for civil servants, prisoners, members of high-risk groups and foreigners seeking residence (other than citizens of Western European countries). In early 1988 Frankfurt city council reported as seeking "remand for treatment under medical supervision" of eight women and two men who were all continuing to practise prostitution despite previous legal injunctions [*Le Monde*, Paris, 5 January 1988].

GREECE
First reported case: 1983
Cases reported March 1988: 106 (11 per million)
Breakdown: At December 1987: 47% homosexual contact, 24% blood product recipient, 23% heterosexual contact, 1% ivdu, 1% homosexual/ivdu, 3% other/undetermined.
Seropositivity: In 1986: 0.02% of blood donors, 45% of haemophiliacs, 3.4% of prostitutes, 2.1% among drug addicts [GDSR, June 1986]. 1987: 12/434 (2.8%) ivdus, 8/623 (1.3%) imprisoned ivdus [A. Roumeliotou et al, SICA II, p192].
Action: STP endorsed January 1988.

The national education campaign has included mailing a leaflet to every household.

HUNGARY
First reported case: 1986
Cases reported May 1988: 12 (1 per million)
Breakdown: at December 1987: 63% homosexual contact, 25% blood product recipients, 13% heterosexual contact.
Seropositivity: To September 1987: total of 139 individuals. Seventy-four of the first 107

people discovered seropositive were homosexual [NS, 12 March 1987].
Compulsory testing: partners of those infected, individuals testing for STDs, individuals charged with prostitution offences, intravenous drug users.

General consensus that AIDS is being approached with a more tolerant attitude than in neighbouring countries. Official recognition (the first in Eastern Europe) given to a national organisation of homosexual men and women in June 1988. While confidentiality is guaranteed for those discovered to be HIV+, the authorities "will take necessary measures" with those who fail to follow doctors' instructions [MTI press release, 10 June 1988]. Transfusion blood reported screened since 1986.

ICELAND
First reported case: 1986
Cases reported May 1988: 5 (25 per million)
Breakdown: First 4 cases all homosexual men.
Seropositivity: To January 1988: 13.5% of homosexuals, 2.9% of ivdus, 0.9% of heterosexuals, 1/23,306 (0.04%) blood donations. Total of 35 identified out of estimated total of 200-400 (0.1%- 0.2% of the population) [HMC].
Action: AIDS Advisory Committee set up in 1986. Assessment visit completed.
Internal regulations: quarantine reported (see below).

In May 1987 a woman was reportedly placed under house arrest because of "irresponsible sexual conduct" [GDSR, Aug 1987]. Transfusion blood screened since 1985.

IRELAND
First reported case: 1985
Cases reported May 1988: 37 (11 cases per million).
Breakdown: at December 1987: 37% homosexual contact, 30% ivdu, 17% blood product recipients, 13% homosexual/ivdu, 3% heterosexual contact.
Seropositivity: In February 1988: 24% of drug users, 25% of haemophiliacs, 6% of homo/bisexuals; total of 678 identified, 60% of whom between 15 and 24 years old [G. Dean, GIA, p40].

With 35 infants born with the virus, Ireland has highest incidence of HIV-positive babies per capita in Europe [*Scotsman*, Edinburgh, 15 February 1988]. A large number of prisoners reported to be seropositive, with an isolation unit in Mountjoy Prison for those carrying the virus. Close economic and social ties with the neighbouring United Kingdom may be contributing to the spread of AIDS. In early 1988 the *Irish Times* reported that four out of ten patients at the St Mary's Drug Dependence Unit in London were from Dublin [*Scotsman*, Edinburgh, 15 February 1988].

ITALY
First reported case: June 1982
Cases reported April 1988: 1,865 (32 per million)
Breakdown at December 1987: 64% ivdu, 21% homosexual contact, 4% blood product recipients, 4% homosexual contact/ivdu, 4% heterosexual contact, 3% others/undetermined. See also below.
Seropositivity: To March 1988: estimated as 27.5 people HIV+ for each person with AIDS [G. Luzi et al, GIA, p 59.], implying total of 40,000 (0.07% of the population). HIV-2 detected in 3/328 sera (all 3 non-Italians) [O. E. Varnier, SICA II, p223].

In the first half of 1984 62.5% of new AIDS cases were homosexual men, 25% drug users. Heterosexual contact first confirmed as a means of transmission in the first half of 1986; almost 50% of all AIDS cases in Lombardy, which includes the city of Milan. Numbers there are three times as high as the next-affected region, Lazio, which encompasses Rome, [*Babilonia*, Milan, December 1987 & January/February 1988]. There has been some controversy as to whether the country is reacting sufficiently to the AIDS epidemic. The head of the Italian AIDS commission was dismissed in February 1988, reportedly for criticising the Minister of Health for lack of funds to fight the epidemic [*La Repubblica*, Rome, 25 February 1988; *Guardian*, London, 26 February 1988]. Another specialist on AIDS, Dr Mauri Moroni, has claimed that educational measures have not been effective and that sales of condoms and syringes have not risen to any great extent [*Babilonia*, Milan, January/February 1988].

LUXEMBOURG
First reported case: 1985
Cases reported May 1988: 10 (25 per million)
Breakdown: first eight cases: 4 homosexual contact, 1 ivdu, 1 blood recipient, 2 unknown.
Seropositivity in 1987: 1/13,000 (0.008%) blood donors.
Action: National AIDS Surveillance Committee set up in 1983.

An education campaign began in March 1987 with a budget of FB7 million (US$190,000). During the ten weeks in which an AIDS hot-line was in operation, it received more than 36,000 calls, equivalent to one-tenth of the population.

MALTA
First reported case: 1986
Cases reported April 1988: 10 (25 per million)
Seropositivity: To January 1988: total of 27 HIV+; the virus was initially seen mostly in haemophiliacs but the trend is moving towards homosexuals [HMC].

MONACO
First reported case: December 1987
Cases reported December 1987: 1 (37 per million)

NETHERLANDS
First reported case: 1982
Cases reported June 1988: 526 (36 per million)
Breakdown: at December 1987: 85.5% homosexual contact, 3.8% ivdu, 2.4% blood product recipients, 1.9% heterosexual contact, 1.4% paediatric, 1.2% homosexual/ivdu, 3.8% unknown; 96.4% male, 3.6% female.
Seropositivity: In 1986: 15/527,000 (0.003%) blood donors [GDSR, November 1987].

NORWAY
First reported case: 1984
Cases reported April 1988: 81 (19 per million)
Breakdown: 74.1% homosexual contact, 11.1% blood product recipients, 8.6% heterosexual contact, 4.9% ivdu, 1.2% unknown; 90.1% male, 9.9% female.
Seropositivity: Mid-1987: estimated 3,000 (0.07% of the population) [GDSR, August 1987]. HIV-2 reported in July 1987.

As part of its education campaign Norway has a successful policy of inviting drug abusers onto local AIDS committees.

POLAND
First reported case: 1986
Cases reported May 1988: 3 (0.08 per million)
Seropositivity: December 1987: 55/400,000 (0.01%) blood tests, the majority believed at high risk [GDSR, January 1988]. To June 1988: 0/20,189 blood donors [P. Boron et al, SICA I, p304].

Entry restrictions: Foreign students.

Education campaign launched in March 1988; the use of condoms urged despite church opposition and a shortage of contraceptives [*Independent*, London, 24 March 1988].

PORTUGAL

First reported case: 1983
Cases reported May 1988: 125 (12 per million)
Breakdown: At December 1987: 50.0% homosexual contact, 36.7% heterosexual contact/undetermined, 8.9% haemophiliac, 4.4% ivdu; 90% male, 10% female.
Seropositivity: In 1986: 15/84,932 (0.02%) blood donations. In 1987: 9% of drug abusers, 25% of homo/bisexual men. [CP] HIV-2 much less common than HIV-1; a higher proportion of homosexual men than prostitutes are infected [J. Cardoso et al, GIA, p27.].

ROMANIA

First reported case: 1985
Cases reported April 1988: 4 (0.2 per million)
Seropositivity: To August 1987: 13 individuals of unidentified risk status. [NS, 20 August 1987].

An AIDS prevention campaign had not been announced by June 1988. If launched, it is likely to conflict with the official government policy of banning all forms of contraceptives in order to encourage population growth.

SAN MARINO

No cases of AIDS reported.
Seropositivity: 1986/7: 7 HIV+ (0.03% of the total population), 0/2,560 blood donations (one-twelfth of the population) positive [HMC].

SPAIN

First reported case: 1981
Cases reported April 1988: 1,126 (29 per million)
Breakdown: at December 1987: 52% intravenous drug use, 24% homosexual contact, 10% blood product recipients, 6% homosexual/ivdu, 2% children of parent at risk, 1% heterosexual contact, 5% undetermined; 86% male, 14% female.
Seropositivity: January 1988: estimated at 100,000 (0.3% of the population) [HMC]. 1987: 49.3% of 478 ivdus, 10.6% of 123 homosexual men [V. Cárcaba et al, SICA I, p300]. 55% of 307 male prisoners, 26% of 95 female prisoners in Madrid [P. Estebanez, SICA I, p311] (see below).
Action: National AIDS Working Commission founded in May 1983.

The doubling rate for AIDS cases slowed from 7.3 months at the end of 1986 to 14.7 months at the end of 1987. In Catalonia, in N. E. Spain, the major route of transmission is homosexual contact. HIV infection reported widespread in Spanish jails, with 30% of inmates in Carabanchel prison, Madrid, seropositive [*Independent*, London, 13 May 1987]. In an incident in southern Spain prisoners held guards hostage to demand free syringes and condoms [*Independent*, London, 27 April 1987]. A special prison programme has been set up under the AIDS prevention campaign and includes training of prison health personnel and distribution of condoms.

SWEDEN

First reported case: 1983
Cases reported June 1988: 197 (23 per million)
Breakdown: At July 1987: 96.2% male, 3.8% female. At December 1987: 81% homosexual contact, 12% blood product recipients, 7% heterosexual contact.

Seropositivity: To December 1987: total of 1,007 [GDSR, January 1988], 50/350 (14%) drug abusers [GDSR, December 1987].
Internal restrictions: Law permits indefinite isolation of persons with contagious diseases (see Chapter Nine).

Majority of people with AIDS/HIV in Stockholm; Malmö the next most infected area. In 1988 the Swedish Red Cross Society entered into partnership with the NGO Ark of Noah to launch an integrated community-based programme of support, shelter, counselling and information for people with AIDS and HIV. A building in central Stockholm houses an AIDS hotline, drop-in and counselling facilities, information database and temporary residential accommodation for PWAs in crisis.

SWITZERLAND
First reported case: 1981
Cases reported March 1988: 439 (67 per million)
Breakdown: At December 1987: 61.4% homosexual contact, 18.3% ivdu, 10.0% heterosexual contact, 3.0% homosexual/ivdu, 1.3% blood product recipient, 2.0% paediatric, 4.0% undetermined; 83% male, 17% female.
Seropositivity: To January 1988: estimated at 20,000-30,000 (0.3%-0.4% of the population) [HMC]; this figure includes 50% of ivdus, 15% of homosexual men and 0.1%-0.5% child-bearing women [J. Osterwalder et al, SICA I, p302].

Between June 1986 and December 1987 the percentage of women with AIDS rose from 10% to 17% while the percentage of men and women with a history of drug abuse rose from 14% to 21%.

USSR
First reported case: 1986
Cases reported March 1988: 4 (0.01 per million). 1 Soviet Citizen (see below), 3 Africans.
Seropositivity: To March 1988: 240 foreigners (all since deported), 47 Soviet citizens of 3.7 million blood tests (including 120,000 to 150,000 people at high risk, the rest blood donors). This 47 includes 16 prostitutes connected with the Soviet citizen with AIDS (see below), 10-12 prostitutes who had had sexual relations with foreigners, 6 homosexuals, 1 woman who injected drugs [V. Pokrovsky, speaking at GIA]. HIV-2 not identified but health authorities reported searching for the virus [*Nature*, 3 December 1987].
Action: Assessment visit completed.
Entry restrictions: Long-term visitors.
Internal regulations: Foreigners and citizens subject to testing on demand; isolation permitted by law.

The Soviet citizen with AIDS was an interpreter who had spent some time in Tanzania. As well as the 16 prostitutes mentioned above his infection has spread to five other Soviet citizens. One of the latter gave blood, from which five further cases of HIV infection resulted, including two infants. As part of the continuing campaign against AIDS the existence of drug abuse and homosexuality in the USSR has been officially recognised [*Libération*, Paris, 17 February 1988]. One major problem facing the country is a shortage of condoms; in early 1988 a British businessman, Richard Branson, was negotiating the export of his company's condoms to the Soviet Union.

UNITED KINGDOM
First reported case: 1982
Cases reported May 1988: 1,541 (27 per million)
Breakdown: 83.0% homosexual contact, 8.3% blood product recipients, 3.4% heterosexual contact, 1.8% ivdu, 1.6% homosexual/ivdu, 1.0% child of parent at risk, 0.8% undetermined.
Seropositivity: To March 1988: 8,443 discovered, total estimated at 30,000-100,000 (0.05-0.18% of the population). Very high rates (up to 50%) among drug users in Scotland,

particularly Edinburgh, where 1,000 heroin users and 15% of their sexual partners were estimated HIV-positive [*Times*, London, 20 February 1988]. 30% of ivdus at one London clinic were HIV-positive at March 1987.

Intravenous drug usage is on the increase in the UK and treatment facilities are inadequate. The wide-ranging government campaign linking the injection of drugs with AIDS was criticised by Afro-Caribbean and Asian AIDS activists for ignoring their communities.

YUGOSLAVIA
First reported case: 1985
Cases reported March 1988: 38 (2 per million).
Breakdown: at December 1987: 40% homosexual contact, 28% ivdu, 12% blood product recipients, 8% heterosexual contact, 4% homosexual contact/ivdu, 8% other/unknown.
Seropositivity: In 1987: 700 identified, the majority ivdu. To June 1988: 286/652 (43.9%) ivdus, 27/56 (48.2%) haemophiliacs, 5/76 (6.8%) homosexual men, 8/33 (24.2%) promiscuous heterosexuals, all in Belgrade [Z. Sonja et al, SICA I, p304]; much lower rates in all categories in Zagreb [V. Burek et al, SICA I, p304].

■■■

MIDDLE EAST

REPORTED AIDS CASES at June 1988

	Officially Reported AIDS cases	Population (in millions)	AIDS cases per million population
Qatar	32	.0300	107
Israel	58	4.400	13
Turkey	25	51.400	0.5

These figures exclude countries reporting fewer than 10 cases. Source: Panos, from WHO and national health ministry figures.

Blood screening is carried out in Israel, all Gulf countries and to some extent in other countries. Seroprevalence is generally thought to be low. Education campaigns have been initiated to a greater or lesser extent in almost every country. Entry restrictions have been reported, although not always confirmed, from Kuwait, Saudi Arabia, Qatar, the United Arab Emirates and Yemen. Other Gulf countries may prohibit entry to individuals carrying HIV. Those principally affected are thousands of migrant workers from South-East Asia. In Indonesia, the Philippines, Thailand and other countries in the region, Saudi consular authorities will only accept HIV-negative certificates from medical centres which they have inspected. Applicants for work permits from other countries also have to provide such a certificate. It is understood that certificates must bear the photograph of the individual tested. Only Iraq (see below), requires short-term visitors to be tested.

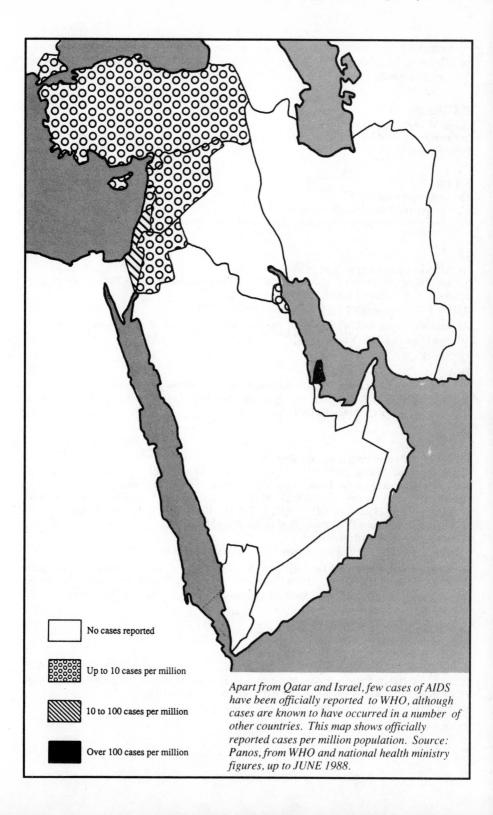

No cases reported

Up to 10 cases per million

10 to 100 cases per million

Over 100 cases per million

Apart from Qatar and Israel, few cases of AIDS have been officially reported to WHO, although cases are known to have occurred in a number of other countries. This map shows officially reported cases per million population. Source: Panos, from WHO and national health ministry figures, up to JUNE 1988.

Reminder: Seropositivity studies of a specific segment of a population (eg prostitutes or blood donors in a large city) should **not** be taken as representative of the country as a whole.

BAHRAIN
No AIDS cases reported by June 1988.
Seropositivity: Mid-1987: Eleven Bahrainis, including three drug users, reported HIV-positive [GDSR, August 1987].

CYPRUS
First reported case: 1986
Cases reported June 1987: 3 (4 per million).
Entry restrictions: foreigners seeking work in cabarets/night clubs; African students.

IRAN
No AIDS cases reported by May 1988.
Seropositivity: In 1986: 10/100 haemophiliacs, 0/505 others at risk HIV-positive [*Weekly Epidemiological Record*, WHO, 1986, 61(19), 145].
Action: MTP from August 1988, TSA from December 1987.

An unoffical report in 1987 suggested that two people had died of AIDS contracted through infected blood [GDSR, October 1987].

IRAQ
No AIDS cases reported or seroepidemiological studies published by May 1988.
Entry restrictions: All foreigners staying longer than five days (other than diplomats) and all returning Iraqis must be screened for HIV.

ISRAEL
First reported case: 1980 (post diagnosis)
Cases reported March 1988: 58 (13 per million). Majority of reported AIDS cases in homosexual men and haemophiliacs; only one of first 45 cases (2.2%) ivdu.
Seropositivity: To January 1988: 300 identified HIV+, including 55 (18.3%) ivdus; 10/300,000 (0.003%) donated blood units HIV+ [HMC]. To June 1988: 7/52 (6.9%) male prisoners, 3/113 (2.7%) female prisoners [E. Rubinstein et al, SICA I, p312].
Action: Assessment visit completed.
Internal regulations: Prostitutes are required to be tested every six months.

A cheap alternative treatment for AIDS, which aims to prevent the virus replicating, has been developed in Israel. Called AL-721 and based on egg extracts, it has achieved some success in trials in both Israel and the United States. Transfusion blood screened since April 1986.

JORDAN
First reported case: 1987
Cases reported December 1987: 3 (0.8 per million)
Seropositivity: Mid-1987: 12 HIV+: 8 Jordanians and 4 foreigners [GDSR, October 1987]; 9/21,727 (0.0004%) blood donors tested at central blood bank and the University Hospital HIV+ [report by National Committee on AIDS and WHO, August 1987].
Action: MTP planned or ongoing, TSA from December 1987.
The government has issued leaflets about AIDS.

KUWAIT
First reported case: December 1987 (see below)
Cases reported December 1987: 1 (0.5 per million)
Seropositivity: 1986-87: "few" of 100,000 samples, mostly blood product related [K. Behbehani et al, SICA II, p269].
Action: National Committee set up in 1985: assessment visit completed.
Entry restrictions: residence and work permit applicants.

A transfusion-related case was unofficially reported in early 1986 [NS, 30 Jan 1986]. The government has launched an education campaign. Transfusion blood screened since 1985.

OMAN
No AIDS cases reported or seroepidemiological studies published by June 1988.
Action: National AIDS Committee formed in July 1986; assessment visit planned.

Donated blood has been screened since July 1986.

QATAR
First reported case: May 1987
Cases reported December 1987: 32 (107 per million). At least seven cases are blood product recipients.
Entry restrictions: Residence and work permit applicants.

SAUDI ARABIA
No AIDS cases reported to WHO by June 1988, although according to one source "18 persons had contracted the virus" of whom 7 had died [IHT, 21 March 1988].
Seropositivity: 1986-88: 5/23,000 (0.02%) blood donors [A.M. Al Rasheed et al, SICA I, p315].
Entry restrictions: "People coming to work from certain countries".

All donated blood now screened.

SYRIA
First reported case: October 1986
Cases reported August 1987: 5 (0.4 per million)
Breakdown: 4 Syrian, 1 Tanzanian; 4 male, 1 female; 1 blood product recipient, 2 heterosexual contact, 1 child of parent at risk, 1 undetermined.
Seropositivity: 0/473 blood donors, 0/240 male prisoners, 0/145 female "entertainers", 0/200 health service workers, 0/87 foreign workers and 0/2442 patients diagnosed with non-AIDS illnesses [CP].
Action: MTP planned, TSA from December 1987.
Entry restrictions: Work permit applicants; foreign students.

An AIDS education campaign began in 1986 with information aimed primarily at health workers and foreign travellers. A school education campaign is under discussion.

TURKEY
First reported case: November 1985
Cases reported September 1987: 25 (0.5 per million)
Breakdown: 36% blood product recipients, 24% homosexual contact/ivdu, 8% heterosexual contact, 32% undetermined; 84% male, 16% female.
Seropositivity: To February 1987: 12 individuals identified HIV+ [GDSR, February 1987].

UNITED ARAB EMIRATES
No AIDS cases reported by May 1988, although one source announced a transfusion-related case early in 1986 [NS, 30 January 1986].
Action: Assessment visit planned.
Entry restrictions: Work permit applicants.

YEMEN (NORTH)
No AIDS cases reported or seroepidemiological studies published by May 1988.
Action: STP drawn up.

YEMEN, PEOPLE'S DEMOCRATIC REPUBLIC (SOUTH)
No cases of AIDS reported or epidemiological studies published by May 1988. In October 1987 it was reported that three HIV+ foreigners were identified and deported [GDSR, October 1987].
Action: MTP from March 1988, TSA from October 1987.

■■

AFRICA

Reminder: Seropositivity studies of a specific segment of a population (eg prostitutes or blood donors in a large city) should **not** be taken as representative of the country as a whole.

REPORTED AIDS CASES at June 1988

	Officially reported AIDS cases	Population (in millions)	AIDS cases per million population
Congo	1,250	2.10	595
Burundi	1,156	5.00	231
Uganda	2,369	15.90	149
Rwanda	901	6.80	133
Zambia	754	7.10	106
Central Afr Rep	254	2.70	94
Malawi	583	7.400	79
Tanzania	1,608	23.50	68
Kenya	1,497	22.40	67
Gambia	35	0.80	44
Ivory Coast	250	10.80	23
Guinea-Bissau	16	0.90	18
Gabon	18	1.150	16
Botswana	16	1.20	13
Zimbabwe*	119	9.40	13
Zaire	335	31.80	11
Ghana	145	13.90	10
Senegal	66	7.10	9

Cameroon	47	10.30	5
Tunisia	30	7.60	4
Burkina Faso	26	7.30	4
South Africa	120	34.30	4
Mali	29	8.40	3
Angola	23	8.00	3
Sudan	35	23.50	1
Morocco	14	21.90	0.6
Ethiopia	35	46.00	0.8
Algeria	13	23.50	0.6
Nigeria	11	108.60	0.1

The above figures exclude countries reporting fewer than 10 cases. Source: Panos, from WHO and national health ministry figures.

*In April 1988, Zimbabwe withdrew its earlier reported figure of 380 cases pending a national review of the accuracy of the reporting system [*Weekly Epidemiological Record*, 6 May 1988, p138]. Other countries where an earlier reported figure has been higher than those given in this document include Nicaragua, Paraguay and the USSR.

ALGERIA
First reported case: 1986
Cases reported April 1988: 13 (0.6 per million)
Seropositivity: Total of 90 HIV+ identified; 18% of haemophiliacs HIV+ [*Jeune Afrique*, 1 June 1988].
Action: STP endorsed January 1988.

An unofficial source gives 60 AIDS cases by May 1988. Workers returning from abroad are said to have to undergo an HIV-antibody test [*Jeune Afrique*, 1 June 1988].

ANGOLA
First reported case: 1985
Cases reported December 1987: 23 (3 per million)
Breakdown: First four AIDS cases in Europeans, one from blood transfusion, three from heterosexual contact.
Seropositivity: To June 1987: 2/452 (0.4%) male blood donors, 1/357 (0.3%) pregnant women, 1/100 (1%) tuberculosis patients, 4/94 (4%) hospital patients [B. Böttiger et al, WICA, p176]. 27 HIV+ individuals identified by the end of 1987, male:female ratio of 1:1; the north of the country is worst affected [HMC]. To June 1988: 10% of 563 non-patients and 22% of 621 patients (including STDs and TB) HIV-1+, HIV-2+ or HIV-1/-2+ [M. O. Santos Ferreira et al, SICA I, p325].
Action: MTP from June 1988, TSA from December 1987.

BENIN
First reported case: 1986
Cases reported December 1987: 9 (2 per million)
Seropositivity: To January 1987: 0/1,286 blood donors, 0/878 pregnant women, 7/215 (3%) prostitutes [D. Latinne et al, AACIA, p82]. In May 1987: of 133 female prostitutes 6 (4.5%) HIV-1+, 5 (3.7%) HIV-2+ (10 of the 11 non-Beninois); 4/334 (1.2%) soldiers and patients HIV-1+, 1/200 (0.5%) prisoners HIV-2+; 0/256 male prostitutes, health workers, pregnant women and blood donors HIV- 1+ or HIV-2+ [I. Zohoun et al, SICA I, p330].
Action: MTP from June 1988, TSA from August 1987.

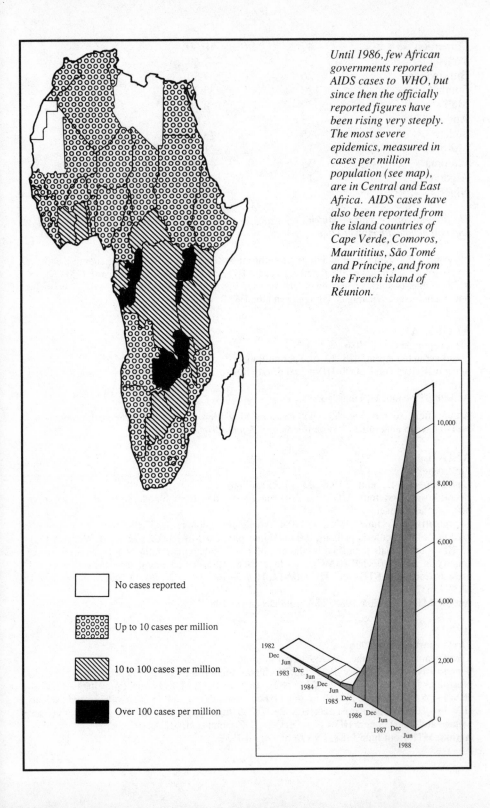

*Until 1986, few African
governments reported
AIDS cases to WHO, but
since then the officially
reported figures have
been rising very steeply.
The most severe
epidemics, measured in
cases per million
population (see map),
are in Central and East
Africa. AIDS cases have
also been reported from
the island countries of
Cape Verde, Comoros,
Maurititius, São Tomé
and Príncipe, and from
the French island of
Réunion.*

No cases reported

Up to 10 cases per million

10 to 100 cases per million

Over 100 cases per million

10,000

8,000

6,000

4,000

2,000

0

1982
Dec
Jun
1983 Dec
Jun
1984 Dec
Jun
1985 Dec
Jun
1986 Dec
Jun
1987 Dec
Jun
1988

BOTSWANA
First reported case: 1986
Cases reported January 1988: 16 (13 per million)
Seropositivity: To mid-1987: 27/6,000 (0.5%) tests (inc. 5,500 blood donors) [C. J. van Dam, personal communication]. To June 1988: 11/257 (4.3%) hospital patients [W.D. Osei et al, SICA I, p329].
Action: MTP completed July 1987.

Eleven of first 13 AIDS cases were Botswana citizens, the majority women. An education campaign began in March 1987. Botswana's national AIDS committee is broadly composed and contains several non-scientists.

BURKINA FASO
First reported case: 1987
Cases reported June 1987: 26 (4 per million)
Seropositivity: To 1987: 3.1% HIV-1, 7.7% HIV-2, of 779 sera [L. Sangare et al, AACIA, p81]. To June 1988: of hospitalised patients 23% HIV-1+ and 0.5% HIV-2+ [R. Soudre, SICA I, p322].
Action: MTP from August 1988, TSA from 1987.

BURUNDI
First reported case: 1984
Cases reported June 1988: 1,156 (231 per million). 54% male, 46% female.
Seropositivity: To 1986: 12/65 (18%) STD patients, 4/93 (4%) non-STD patients in one rural area [M. Galli et al, AACIA, p90]. Mid-1987: 6% of blood donors in/around Bujumbura [HMC].
Action: MTP ongoing, TSA from August 1987.

CAMEROON
First reported case: 1986
Cases reported March 1988: 47 (5 per million). 45% male, 55% female.
Seropositivity: To June 1987: 11/1,761 (0.6%) adults, 10 (3 Cameroonian)/358 (2.8%) hospitality girls; in Yaoundé and Nkongsamba 0/319 children under 15, 0/488 outpatients. [J. P. Durand et al, WICA, p123]. In late 1987: reckoned as 2% in Douala [GDSR, December 1987]. HIV-2 has been reported [R.C. Kooiman et al, GIA, p26]. To June 1988: 0/370 healthy adults, 0/119 patients, 4/53 (7.5%) prostitutes and 1/35 (2.9%) prisoners HIV-1+ [K. Youkokuda et al, SICA I, p351].
Action: MTP completed, TSA from June 1987. A government education campaign began in January 1987.

CAPE VERDE
First reported case: 1985
Cases reported April 1987: 4 (·13 per million).
Seropositivity: To June 1987: 9/110 (8%) prisoners, 2/93 (2%) soldiers, 2/13 (15%) blood donors, 2/2 women with AIDS all HIV- 2+, none HIV-1+ [F. Brun-Vezinet et al, WICA, p211].
Action: STP completed, TSA from December 1987.

CENTRAL AFRICAN REPUBLIC
First reported case: 1984
Cases reported October 1986: 254 (94 per million).
Seropositivity: October 1984-January 1987: 2.1-4.0% of general population, 12.0-20.6% of hospitality girls [A. J. Georges et al, WICA, p123]. Seropositivity rose from 2.5% in 1985 to 7.8% in March 1987 [*Lancet*, 1987, ii (December 5), 1,332-3]. HIV-2 detected [F. Schon & J.

Blau, *Lancet*, 23 January 1988].
Action: MTP completed, TSA from August 1987.

Non-WHO source reported 587 AIDS cases [*Lancet*, 1987, ii (December 5), p1,332-3].

CHAD
First reported case: 1986
Cases reported November 1986: 1 (0.2 per million)
Seropositivity: To 1986: 0.3% (+/- 0.6%) of 331 sera in Njamena in 1986 [M.C. Georges-Courbot et al, AACIA, p86].
Action: MTP to start August 1988.

COMOROS
First reported case: 1988
Cases reported May 1988: 1 (2 per million)
Seropositivity: March-December 1987: 0/239 STD patients, 0/98 tuberculosis patients, 0/239 military recruits HIV+ [E. Petat et al, SICA II, p242].

CONGO
First reported case: 1983
Cases reported December 1987: 1,250 (595 per million).
Seropositivity: October 1986-September 1987: 1,005/13,505 (7.4%) HIV+ according to ELISA; 477 tests available for Western Blot, of which 220 were confirmed positive [N. Copin et al, SICA I, p347]. February-April 1987: 23/67 (34%) Brazzaville prostitutes HIV+ according to ELISA [P. M'Pele et al, AACIA, p87].
Action: National AIDS Committee set up in 1985; MTP completed, TSA from August 1987.

One in three patients at Adolphe Sice Hospital in Pointe Noire and 15 to 20 new patients a month at Makelele Hospital, Brazzaville reported with AIDS [IHT, 23-24 January 1988]. Transfused blood is screened for 80% of the population.

DJIBOUTI
No cases of AIDS reported by June 1988.
Seropositivity: In October 1987: "weak" incidence of infection [HMC]. In late 1987: 8/645 (2 men, 6 female prostitutes) (1.2%) [E. A. Abbatte, SICA I, p327].
Action: The government has approached WHO and the European Community for aid in instigating a short-term plan [HMC]. MTP planned.

EGYPT
First reported case: July 1987
Cases reported January 1988: 5 (0.1 per million).
Seropositivity: 1986-87: 16/10,234 samples (0.16%), including blood product recipients and international travellers [F. Sheba et al, SICA I, p316]. To June 1988: 0/20,000 samples (including 15,000 at high risk) [M. I. Shaker et al, SICA I, p315].
Action: STP ongoing.

EQUATORIAL GUINEA
No cases of AIDS reported by June 1988.
Seropositivity: In 1985: 0.3% (+/-0.6%) of 308 sera in Bioco [M.C. Georges-Courbot et al, AACIA, p86].
Action: STP planned.

ETHIOPIA
First reported case: 1987
Cases reported April 1988: 37   (0.8 per million)
Seropositivity: In 1985-86 4/5,606 (0.07%) mostly military recruits [S. Buttò et al, AACIA, p117].   To June 1987: 4/60 (6.7%) prostitutes, 0/70 prostitutes' clients, 0/230 others [S. Ayehunie, WICA, p45]. To June 1988: 56/869 (6.4%) individuals, including many at high risk [S. Ayehunie, SICA I, p325].
Action: MTP completed, TSA from June 1987.

GABON
First reported case: 1987
Cases reported March 1988: 18   (16 cases per million)
Seropositivity: In 1986: 0% in north, 0.8% in southern rural areas, 1.8% in Libreville [E. Delaporte et al, AACIA, p 86].
Action: MTP from August 1988, TSA from December 1987.

GAMBIA
First reported case: 1987
Cases reported March 1988: 35   (44 per million)
Seropositivity: 10/185 (5.4%) STD patients HIV-2+, 1/278 (0.4%) blood donors HIV-2+, none in either group HIV-1+ [Dept of Health, Banjul, et al, SICA I, p316].
Action: MTP from August 1988, TSA from September 1987.

GHANA
First reported case: May 1986
Cases reported May 1987: 145   (10 per million)
Seropositivity: To late 1987: Total of 276 HIV-1+; in Accra 6/5,480 (0.1%) blood donors (0.1%), 2/300 (0.7%) intending travellers HIV-1+, also 0.7% of prostitutes in 1986 rising to 2.2% in 1987; female:male ratio 11:1 in 1986 and 7.6:1 in 1987 [A. R. Neequaye, presentation at GIA].
Action: National Technical Committee on AIDS established in October 1985; MTP from June 1988, TSA from October 1987.

199 (59.4%) of seropositives are women prostitutes returning from the Ivory Coast with 50%+ of all seropositive cases in the Eastern Region, which has strong links with the Ivory Coast. Decreasing female:male ratio of seropositivity suggests increasing indigenous heterosexual spread.   An innovative AIDS education programme among Accra female prostitutes is in progress.

GUINEA
First reported case: 1987
Cases reported November 1987: 4   (0.6 per million)
Seropositivity: In June 1987: 6/756 (0.8%) HIV-1 infection, 2/756 (0.3%) HIV-2 infection, subjects included hospital patients and health care workers; 0/167 women attending clinics, 0/110 military recruits positive for either virus [C. Katlama et al, WICA, p 176].   Another study has found 0.2% HIV-1 infection and 1.3% HIV-2 infection [K. Kourouma et al, AACIA, p79].
Action: MTP from March 1988, TSA from December 1987.Transfusion blood is screened.

GUINEA-BISSAU
First reported case: 1987
Cases reported November 1987: 16   (18 per million)
Seropositivity: In 1986-87: 47/275 (17%) Ministry of Health workers HIV-2+, 3/275 (1%) HIV-1+; of 236 soldiers 9% HIV-2+ and 1% HIV-1+ [A. Santos Pinto et al, p77, & W. F.

Canas Ferreira, AACIA, p78]. HIV-2 but not HIV-1 infection present in 1980 [P. N. Fultz et al, WICA, p22]. Both viruses endemic in rural areas in November 1985 [F. Antunes et al, WICA, p178]. In 1987 seropositivity ranged from 5.1% of scholarship applicants to 33.3% of prostitutes [C. Mendes Costa et al, SICA I, p317].
Action: MTP from June 1988, TSA from August 1987.

IVORY COAST
First reported case: 1986
Cases reported November 1987: 250 (23 per million)
Seropositivity: In 1986: 2.7% of 850 healthy adults, 6.1% of 350 patients receiving multiple injections, 8.9% of 1,200 individuals with multiple sex partners (all HIV-1) [G. Leonard et al, WICA, p211]. HIV-1 and HIV-2 both endemic [A. Outtara et al, WICA, p88]. To June 1988: of pregnant women 7% HIV-1+, 0.5% HIV-2+; other hospitalised groups with higher rates [K. Odehouri et al, SICA I, p318].
Action: MTP from April 1988, TSA from December 1987.

See also Ghana.

KENYA
First reported case: 1983
Cases reported December 1987: 1,497 (67 per million)
Seropositivity: In 1986/87: 77/2,910 (2.6%) pregnant women in Nairobi, 1/103 hospital patients in rural north-east [J. K. Kreiss et al, p64 & A. Saracco et al, AACIA, p91]. 1.5%-2% of donated blood [*Daily Nation*, Nairobi, 3 February 1988].
Action: MTP completed, TSA from June 1987.

US$2.9 million pledged by foreign donors for the national campaign launched in February 1988; a further US$11.3 million budgeted for following four years [NS, 7 January 1988; *Kenya Times*, 13 February 1988]. Transfusion blood is screened. One of the earliest and best publicised AIDS education programmes with women prostitutes is in progress in Nairobi. The Kenyan Red Cross Society has been very active in AIDS information work.

LESOTHO
First reported case: 1986
Cases reported November 1987: 2 (1 per million
Seropositivity: Between April and June 1987: 0/1,006 blood donors.
Action: MTP complete, TSA from October 1987.

Transfusion blood in Maseru screened since April 1987; hospitals elsewhere may use locally-drawn blood not tested for HIV. Approximately 50% of the total adult male labour force of Lesotho work in South African mines. STD and tuberculosis rates, both possible indicators of HIV risk, are high in this group, with potentially explosive implications for mineworkers and their families. [WHO STP report, Ministry of Health, Lesotho, July 1987]

LIBERIA
First reported case: 1987
Cases reported June 1987: 2 (0.8 per million)
Seropositivity: In 1987: 0/493 blood donors, USA visa applicants and others [C. P. Freeman et al, SICA I, p319].
Action: MTP from 1988, TSA from August 1987.

LIBYA
No AIDS cases reported or seroepidemiological studies published by March 1988.
Action: Assessment visit planned.
Entry restrictions: Foreign students, applicants for "residence for professional purposes".

MADAGASCAR
No AIDS cases reported or seroepidemiological studies published by March 1988.
Action: STP completed.

MALAWI
First reported case: 1986
Cases reported October 1987: 583   (79 per million)
Seropositivity: In 1986: 4/96 (4%) antenatal mothers, 148/265 (56%) female prostitutes, 10/32 (31%) male prisoners [L.G. Gürtler et al, WICA, p179]; 119/3,165 (3.76%) expatriate mineworkers in South Africa [B.A. Brink et al, WICA, p6]. In 1987: 7/85 (8%) pregnant women (up from 2% in 1985) [J. Chiphangwi et al, SICA I, p324].
Action: MTP completed, TSA from October 1987.

MALI
First reported case: 1988
Cases reported January 1988: 29   (3 per million)
Seropositivity: HIV-1 and HIV-2 both present [J. M. Allaire et al, WICA, p23]. April 1987: HIV-1+ rates between 0% in pregnant women and infectious disease patients and 10.4% in prostitutes; HIV-2 rates between 1.1% in pregnant women and 15.2% in gastroenterology patients; infection with both viruses at 12.6% in prostitutes [F. Brun-Vezinet et al, SICA I, p319].
Action: MTP from March 1988, TSA from November 1987.

MAURITANIA
No cases reported to WHO by March 1988, although one source reports a death from AIDS in November 1987 [GDSR, December 1987].
Seropositivity: 0.6% of 356 samples at an unknown date [S. M'Boup et al, AACIA, p74].
Action: STP completed.

MAURITIUS
First reported case: 1987
Cases reported September 1987: 1   (0.9 per million)
Seropositivity: To December 1987 0/1,203 people at high risk, 1/5,458 (0.02%) general population [C. Chan Kam et al, SICA II, p243].
Action: MTP completed, TSA from July 1987.

MOROCCO
First reported case: December 1987
Cases reported May 1988: 14 (0.6 per million)
Seropositivity: May 1988: total of 8 reported [*Jeune Afrique*, 1 June 1988].
Action: Assessment visit planned.
A proposal for a national campaign to reach the general public was reportedly rejected by the Moroccan Parliament on religious grounds [*Jeune Afrique*, 1 June 1988]. As from June 1988 Moroccans returning from abroad will be required to take an HIV antibody test on their return [*Jeune Afrique*, 1 June 1988].

MOZAMBIQUE
First reported case: 1986
Cases reported March 1988: 9   (0.6 per million)
Seropositivity: To January 1988: of 1,485 samples of unknown risk, 2.24 in the north, 0.84% in the centre and 0.94% in the south of the country; 2.9% of 763 refugees from rural areas, 3.2% of 126 STD patients from Maputo; HIV-2 detected in 2 of 3 AIDS cases [HMC]. To June 1988: 0.8% of 2,306 blood donors HIV-1+ [J. Barreto et al, SICA I, p347].

Action: MTP drawn up.

Implementation of the medium term plan is likely to be difficult, because of the civil war which has resulted in 1 million internal refugees and over 300,000 refugees from other countries.

NAMIBIA
First reported case: 1987
Cases reported August 1987: 2 (1 per million).
Seropositivity. To 1987: 33/8,750 (0.38%) unstated sample group, but confirmatory tests apparently not complete [GDSR, August 1987].

NIGER
First reported case: 1987
Cases reported October 1987: 9 (1 per million)
Seropositivity: To 1987: 11/2,463 (0.4%) blood donors, 6/743 (0.8%) prisoners [GDSR, December 1987].
Action: MTP from June 1988, TSA from August 1987.

NIGERIA
First reported case: 1987
Cases reported March 1988: 11 (0.1 per million)
Seropositivity: To November 1987: 16/17,762 (0.1%) blood samples from various groups, including nine reported AIDS cases [HMC]. To June 1988: 1/1,066 (0.01%) inmates of Maiduguri and Calabar prisons [J.O. Chikwem et al, SICA I, p319]; 4/823 (0.5%) female prostitutes from Borno and Cross River states [I. Mohammed et al, SICA I, p350]. (The prostitutes averaged more than 3 clients a day.)
Action: National Expert Advisory Committee on AIDS set up in June 1986; MTP from August 1988, TSA from June 1987.

The minister of health has been forthright about the risk of HIV and AIDS in Nigeria. N1.5 million (US$375, 000) in 1987 and N2.5 million (US$565,000) in 1988 allocated to the Advisory Committee's work. Each of Nigeria's 21 states scheduled to have blood screening facilities by the end of 1988. National education campaign began in November 1987.

REUNION (Overseas Département of France)
First reported case: June 1987
Cases reported February 1988: 2 (3 per million)

RWANDA
First reported case: 1983
Cases reported November 1987: 901 (133 per million)
Seropositivity: To 1985: 17-19% in urban populations. Unofficial sources suggest 1987 rate may be 30%.
Action: MTP completed, TSA from July 1987.

Rwanda's AIDS education campaign is described in Chapter Five. Thirty-five per cent of the first 705 reported cases of AIDS were in children under 15 [A. Ndikuyeze, AACIA, p43].

SÃO TOMÉ & PRINCIPE
First reported case: February 1988
Cases reported February 1988: 1 (10 per million)

SENEGAL
First reported case: 1987

Cases reported December 1987: 66 (9 per million)
Seropositivity: constant 0.1% of various groups HIV-1+; between 0.1% and 45% of different regions and population groups HIV-2+ [S. M'Boup et al, AACIA, p51].
Action: MTP completed, TSA from September 1987.

SEYCHELLES
No AIDS cases reported or seroepidemiological studies published by June 1988.

SIERRA LEONE
No AIDS cases confirmed by June 1988. However a citizen of the country was reportedly deported from the Soviet Union in November 1987 for being HIV-positive and was being held in an isolation ward [GDSR November 1987; *African Concord*, 1 January 1988]. Limited seroprevalence testing has not yet discovered any other individuals carrying the virus.

SOMALIA
No AIDS cases reported by June 1988.
Seropositivity: To late 1986: 0/700 blood donor samples [AIDS, 1987, 1(4), 257-8]. 1986-87: 0/194 STD patients; 1/287 (0.3%) prostitutes [J. Burans et al, SICA II, p253].

SOUTH AFRICA
First reported case: 1982
Cases reported April 1988: 120 (4 per million)
Breakdown at December 1987: 76 cases in S. African citizens; 74 male, 2 female; 72 white, 3 black, 1 coloured; 85.5% homosexual contact, 7.9% blood product recipients, 6.6% heterosexual contact. 22 foreign cases: 11 from Malawi, 8 Zambia, 1 Zaire, 1 Canada, 1 Haiti.
Seropositivity: In 1986: in mineworkers ranged from 0.02% of South Africans to 3.76% of Malawians [B. A. Brink et al, WICA, p6]. In 1987: 6.6% of Malawian mineworkers [A. B. Zwi & D. E. Bachmayer, GIA, p30]. Total of 2,500 mineworkers HIV-positive by April 1988, the majority migrants; rate of 0.04% in indigenous mineworkers [*Guardian*, London, 8 April 1988].
Entry restrictions: Applicants for work permits.
Internal regulations: any citizen or non-citizen may be tested on demand; quarantining of people with HIV is allowed.

One report suggested the first black South African with AIDS was identified in December 1987 [*Independent*, London, 22 December 1987], but a Panos source suggests a much earlier date. In early 1988 the government wished to deport seropositive migrant mineworkers already in the country but the move was being resisted by the employers, the Chamber of Mines. Transfusion blood screening is being implemented. Officially published figures may considerably underestimate the prevalence of HIV among black South Africans. Other than from the Chamber of Mines, official AIDS information for the black population has been scarce.

SUDAN
First reported case: 1987
Cases reported January 1988: 35 (1 per million)
Seropositivity: To June 1988: 0/599 individuals at high risk in Port Sudan [J. Burans et al, SICA I, p316].
Action: MTP planned or ongoing, TSA from November 1987.

SWAZILAND
First reported case: 1986
Cases reported July 1987: 7 (10 per million)
Action: MTP from April 1988, TSA from October 1987.

TANZANIA
First reported case: 1984
Cases reported October 1987: 1,608   (68 per million)
Seropositivity: 1985-87: 0% in Arusha, 14-16% blood donors and pregnant women in the north-west, 35% of single female bar workers in Dar es Salaam [AIDS, 1987, 1(4), 217-21, 223-7]. August 1987: Kagera region (where AIDS in Tanzania was originally diagnosed) 1-10% in rural areas, 43% in urban areas, total sample size 1,063 [K. Nyamuryekunge et al, SICA I, p323]. To June 1988: 0/496 in rural centres in N. Tanzania [W.M.M.M. Nkya et al, SIICA I, p328].
Action: MTP completed, TSA from June 1987.
Increased awareness of the risk of HIV and the use of condoms have been documented.

TOGO
First reported case: 1987
Cases reported December 1987: 2   (0.6 per million)
Seropositivity: To February 1987: 21/68 (31%) prostitutes (only 4 Togolese), 0/100 other Togolese [GDSR, June 1987].
Action: STP completed, TSA from June 1988.

TUNISIA
First reported case: 1986
Cases reported May 1988: 30 (4 per million).
Seropositivity: To October 1987: 3/719 (0.42%) prisoners, 18/30 (60%) individuals with coagulation difficulties, 0/198 female prostitutes and 0/690 "controls" [Y. Gharbi et al, AACIA, p97]. To June 1988: 0.13% of 1,500 blood donors, 1.9% of 373 prostitutes [G. Giraldo et al, SICA I, p324]. May 1988: total of 86 HIV+ identified [*Jeune Afrique*, 1 June 1988].
Action: STP endorsed December 1987.

A ten-year national campaign began in August 1987, including blood screening, an education campaign and special attention paid to risk groups such as students, prisoners and soldiers. The campaign is to be broadened in 1988 [*Jeune Afrique*, 1 June 1988].

UGANDA
First reported case: 1982
Cases reported October 1987: 2,369   (149 per million) Male:female ratio: 1:1.2. 90% cases adult, 10% children under 5.
Seropositivity: 1985-1987: 0% children/old people, 15-21% blood donors, 32% long-distance drivers/drivers' mates, 68% barmaids in Lyantonde in South West Uganda [AIDS, 1987, 1(4), 217-21, 223-7]. October 1985-February 1987 in one Kampala antenatal clinic seropositivity rose from 10.6% to 24.1% [Panos source]. August 1987: 490/4,000 (12.2%) randomly selected adults in Mpigi district [J. K. Konde-Lule & E. E. Rwakaikara, SICA I, p324]. To June 1988 20% of pregnant women [G. Giraldo, SICA I, p324].
Action: MTP completed, TSA from March 1987.

AIDS cases reported as 4,001 with deaths from AIDS in the Rakai district more than 60 a week [*Daily Telegraph*, London, 6 June 1988 & *Independent*, London, 7 June 1988]. Ugandan health authorities recognise a serious AIDS crisis in the country, but are responding in the context of a decimated health delivery system and other endemic diseases with high mortality. They seek to improve health provision on all fronts while responding urgently to the spread of HIV.

ZAIRE
First reported case: 1983
Cases reported June 1987: 335 (11 per million)
Seropositivity: In 1987: 7-8% general urban population, 0.5-1% in countryside; in Kinshasa

1% outpatient children, 16% blood donations and 25-40% hospitalised patients [confidential report received by Panos]. 17% in military [GDSR, August 1987]. Rise of 3% in general population per year estimated [Agence France-Presse, *Le Soleil*, Dakar, 24 March 1988].
Action: MTP completed, TSA from March 1987.

AIDS cases have been reported in medical journals since 1983, figures only sent to WHO in 1987. HIV infection found in three deaths in University Hospital, Kinshasa [A. M. Nelson et al, SICA I, p323]. Average funeral and wake costs are US$320, while the average salary is US$30 a month. Hospital and burial costs are paid by the employer but in cases of unemployment the burden generally falls on relatives [F. Davachi et al, GIA, p36].

ZAMBIA
First reported case: 1986
Cases reported April 1988: 754 (106 per million)
Seropositivity: In Lusaka in 1985, 189/1,078 (17.5%) hospital patients, ranging from 8.7% antenatal women to 29% STD patients [M. Melbye et al, *Lancet*, 15 November 1986, pp1113-5]. In the Copperbelt, 13% blood donors, 10% antenatal mothers, 44.4% female patients at a Kitwe hospital [*Daily Telegraph*, London, 6 October 1987] .
Action: MTP completed, TSA from March 1987.

Blood has been screened nationwide since mid-1987; 100,000 donations are made annually [Ministry of Health, Zambia, SICA II, p269].

ZIMBABWE
First reported case: 1983
Cases reported August 1987: 119 (13 per million) (but see note at beginning of section)
Seropositivity: In June 1987: 18.5% at a Harare STD clinic [GDSR, August 1987]. Total of 250,000 people (2.7% of the population) estimated HIV+ by health ministry [GDSR, January 1988; *New African*, London, March 1988].
Action: MTP from March 1988, TSA from November 1987.
Transfusion blood is screened.

···-

SOUTH AND EAST ASIA

While the number of reported AIDS cases in Asia is relatively low, it is rising, and concern in the region has prompted some governments to propose quarantine and mandatory testing (see Chapter Nine).

The First International Conference on AIDS and other sexually transmitted diseases in Asia, held in the Philippines in November 1987, attracted 500 delegates — despite the uncertain political situation — who wrestled with the impact of AIDS in the region. Speakers identified the cultural reluctance to openly discuss sexual behaviour as a challenge to AIDS education. Underreporting remains a problem: due to lack of diagnostic facilities, and perhaps the fear of some governments that accurate reporting would damage the tourist industry.

Reminder: Seropositivity studies of a specific segment of a population (eg prostitutes or blood donors in a large city) should *not* be taken as representative of the country as a whole.

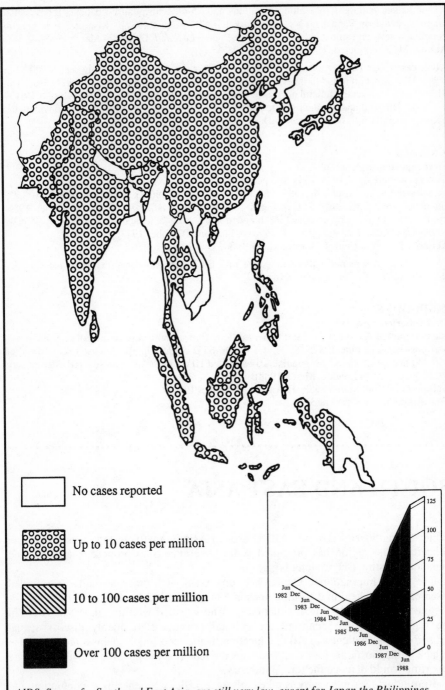

No cases reported

Up to 10 cases per million

10 to 100 cases per million

Over 100 cases per million

AIDS figures for South and East Asia are still very low, except for Japan the Philippines and Thailand, but are growing rapidly, especially among prostitutes. Source: Panos, from WHO and national health ministry figures, up to June 1988.

REPORTED AIDS CASES at June 1988

	Officially reported AIDS cases	Population (in millions)	AIDS cases per million population
Japan	66	122.0	0.5
Thailand	12	53.5	0.2
Philippines	13	61.5	0.2

This table excludes countries reporting fewer than 10 cases. Source: Panos, from WHO and national health ministry figures.

AFGHANISTAN
No AIDS cases reported or seroepidemiological studies published by May 1988.
Action: STP endorsed October 1987, TSA from December 1987.

BANGLADESH
No AIDS cases reported by June 1988.
Seropositivity: None of 10,000 travellers, prisoners, prostitutes and other "vulnerable groups" HIV+ [HMC].
Action: Initial visit ended February 1988.

The greatest risk to Bangladesh comes from "visiting soldiers and sailors". Dirty syringes are also a problem, since they also transmit other diseases, eg. Hepatitis B. Sex is therefore "the least important factor in a country like Bangladesh, because of Bangladesh's moral, spiritual and other attitudes" [HMC].

BHUTAN
No AIDS cases reported or seroepidemiological studies published by June 1988.

BRUNEI
No cases reported by June 1988.
Seropositivity: Unofficially reported in late 1987 as 0.05% [GDSR, January 1988].

Education campaign aimed at the general public began in July 1987.

BURMA
No AIDS cases reported by March 1988.
Seropositivity: September 1985: 0/35 homosexuals, 0/63 prostitutes, 0/16 habitual drug users in Rangoon [GDSR, July 1986].
Action: Initial visit ended February 1988.

CAMBODIA
No AIDS cases reported or seroepidemiological studies published by March 1988.

CHINA
First reported case: 1985
Cases reported December 1987: 3 (0.003 per million) (see below)
Seropositivity: To January 1988: 10/10,000 (0.1%) individuals at high risk, 3 Chinese (all haemophiliac), 7 foreigners [HMC]. To June 0/583 adult blood, 0/95 fetal cord blood in

Sichuan [Q-N Wang et al, SICA II, p245].
Action: Assessment visit.
Entry restrictions: Visitors staying longer than one year; HIV+ tourists deported.
Internal regulations: Chinese returning from abroad are tested; sexual relations with foreigners reportedly forbidden.

The three cases currently reported comprise an Argentinian tourist, a Chinese national who lived in Hong Kong and the USA and a 13-year old haemophiliac infected by imported Factor VIII, all of whom have since died. According to delegate at the health ministers' conference in London, January 1988, "Chinese law and traditional values prohibit homosexuality, sexual promiscuity and the abuse of drug injection [*Guardian*, London, 28 January 1988]." However, it was admitted that there had been a marked increase in STDs in China, blamed on the rising number of western visitors. Research into AIDS prevention and treatment has been incorporated into China's seventh five-year plan (1986-1990), with 300,000 yuan (US$78,000) already allocated. Traditional medicine, including herbal treatment and acupuncture, is a key part of this approach.

CHINA (TAIWAN)
First reported case: 1986
Cases reported January 1986: 1 (0.05 per million) (see below)
Seropositivity: To November 1987: 31 haemophiliac, 17 homosexual, 6 others [M.L. Tan *Report on First International Conference on AIDS in Asia*, November 1987,].

One report suggests a total of 3 AIDS patients and 4 with ARC/PGL to June 1988 [C-Y Chuang & C. H. Chuang, SICA II, p245]. Transfusion blood screened on a sample basis since 1986.

HONG KONG
First reported case: 1985
Cases reported by April 1988: 12 (2 per million).
Seropositivity: April 1985-December 1987: total of 106, including 9/68,643 (0.013%) STD clinic attenders and female prostitutes, 51/137 (37.2%) haemophiliacs, 37 homosexual men [E. K. Yeoh et al, SICA II, p246].

The Hong Kong education campaign began in 1985; the budget for 1986-87 was HK$350,000 (US$45,000). All aspects of the media have been used, in both Chinese and English. Hong Kong's 38,000 drug addicts appear free of infection. Three factors apparently responsible: easily available hypodermic syringes, preference to inhalation not injection of heroin, and narcotics treatment programme which provides methadone at a nominal charge to registered addicts. Currently 9,000 individuals enrolled [IHT, 18 June 1987]. Transfusion blood screened since August 1985.

INDIA
First reported case: 1986
Cases reported May 1987: 9 (0.01 per million).
Seropositivity: Total of 200 individuals HIV+, majority in southern state of Tamil Nadu [*Nature* 11 February 1988]; mostly female prostitutes [M. L. Tan Report on *First International Conference on AIDS in Asia*, November 1987,]. 0/1,000+ blood donors, 0/200 blood product recipients in Maharashtra and Goa [GDSR, October 1987]. To June 1988: 2/2,310 (0.09%) "promiscuous" heterosexuals [P. Seth et al, SICA II, p240]; 33/1,277 (2.6%) female prostitutes, 20/1,743 (1.1%) male STD patients, 0/1,115 in Tamil Nadu [P. G. Babu et al, SICA II, p241]; 37/831 (4.5%) prostitutes in Madras [S. Solomon et al, SICA II, p241].
Action: Assessment visit.
Entry restrictions: foreigners staying more than one year.

The six women first identified in April 1986 as carrying HIV were placed under surveillance. It was reported that 10 women were detained but released because the courts ruled that the government does not have the power to confine individuals on grounds of HIV-positivity. An AIDS Research Centre has been set up in Madras, capital of Tamil Nadu, to co-ordinate surveillance and epidemiology and carry out virological and immunological studies. It is currently the only facility in India to treat people with AIDS [*Nature* 11 February 1988]. In late 1986 the Health Ministry announced that all foreign students (about 18,000 a year, mostly African) would have to take an HIV-antibody test. This led to the immediate expulsion of a number of students and was met with widespread protest by Africans, who accused the Indian government of racism. Eventually the measure was amended to affect only new students and all tourists staying a minimum of a year in India. [For further information on this subject, see Panos book: *Blaming Others: Prejudice, race and worldwide AIDS*]. Intravenous drug use, with several hundred thousand estimated users, is a possible future route of HIV transmission unless prevention campaigns are mounted. But, thus far, government response to AIDS has been confined largely to seroprevalence research and testing.

INDONESIA
First reported case: 1987
Cases reported April 1987: 1 (0.01 per million)
Seropositivity: Late 1987: fewer than 10 seropositive individuals detected [*Jakarta Post*, 7 October & 7 November 1987]. 1986-87: 0/1,918 pregnant women, majority from Bandung area [R. Vranckx et al, SICA II, p245].
Action: MTP from July 1988.
Entry restrictions: people with AIDS denied entry.

A homosexual Canadian who died in November 1987 was reported as the country's second AIDS case. Transfusion blood not routinely screened.

JAPAN
First reported case: March 1985
Cases reported February 1988: 66 (0.5 per million)
Seropositivity: May 1988: total of 1,038 [NS, 26 May 1988], including at least 248 haemophiliacs [GDSR, January 1988].

Most cases of AIDS are in homosexual men and haemophiliacs. The January 1987 death of a Tokyo prostitute, the country's first woman patient and the first to catch AIDS heterosexually, caused near panic with 150,000 telephone calls in the first 48 hours of operation of Tokyo's AIDS information line. Knowledge of the woman's past sexual relations with at least one European confirmed a general view of AIDS as a "foreign" disease. Notices forbidding entry by foreigners have become common in the red light areas. Japan is the world's foremost user of condoms, accounting for 27% of pre-AIDS global use [*Population Reports*, Series 11, number 6, September/October 1982], which may help slow the spread of HIV infection. Transfusion blood is screened.

KOREA, DEMOCRATIC REPUBLIC (NORTH)
No AIDS cases reported or seroepidemiological studies published by June 1988.

KOREA, REPUBLIC (SOUTH)
First reported case: February 1987
Cases reported April 1988: 3 (0.07 per million)
Seropositivity: To February 1988: 11/80,000 (0.01%) 8 prostitutes, 3 others.
Entry restrictions: Under discussion
Internal regulations: Obligatory HIV-certificates for prostitutes; isolation of "high risk" individuals with HIV.

The government is building an isolation centre for individuals at high risk with HIV infection. Proposal for compulsory screening of all foreign visitors was rejected due to fears of jeopardising the success of the 1988 Olympic Games [*New Scientist*, 4 February 1988].

LAOS
No AIDS cases reported or seroepidemiological studies published by May 1988.

MALAYSIA
First reported case: 1987
Cases reported January 1988: 3 (0.2 per million).
Seropositivity: To August 1987: 2/127,000 (0.002%) HIV+ [GDSR, October 1987]. Total of 15 HIV+ individuals by end of 1987 [GDSR January 1988].
Action: National AIDS Task Force set up in March 1985.

Education campaign aimed at homosexuals, ivdus and prostitutes announced in February 1988. Malaysia has over 120,000 registered drug addicts, with an estimated total of over 400,000 (over 2% of the population) [*Indonesian Observer*, 8 February 1988]. Transfusion blood is screened.

MALDIVES
No cases of AIDS reported to WHO by June 1988. One source says a case was reported in April 1987 [GDSR, July 1987]. No seroepidemiological studies published by March 1988.
Action: Initial visit completed February 1988.

MONGOLIA
No AIDS cases reported or epidemiological studies published by June 1988.
Action: MTP from July 1988, TSA from November 1987.
Entry restrictions: Foreign students.

NEPAL
No AIDS cases reported by June 1988.
Seropositivity: To June 1988: none detected [V. L. Guruva Charya, SICA II, p244].
Action: MTP from September 1988, TSA from December 1987.

Transfusion blood is reportedly screened. An information booklet for the general public has been published and a guideline booklet for medical workers is in preparation [V.L. Guruva Charya, as above].

PAKISTAN
First reported case: December 1987
Cases reported by December 1987: 1 (0.1 per million)
Seropositivity: To June 1988: 4/500 (0.8%) sera (2 "promiscuous" males and the wife and child of one) in Karachi and Lahore [S. Rasheed et al, SICA II, p244].
Action: Assessment visit.

Intravenous drug use is reportedly on the rise in urban areas.

PHILIPPINES
First reported case: 1985
Cases reported by April 1988: 13 (0.2 per million)
Breakdown: At July 1987: 8 homosexual contact, 1 blood product recipient; all cases acquired the infection abroad.
Seropositivity: 61/60,0000 tests (0.1%) (, including 49 "hospitality women" [NS, 28 April 1988].
Entry restrictions: Foreigners staying longer than 6 months; refugees; foreign seamen.
Action: STP drawn up.

The 49 "hospitality workers" are associated with US military bases at Olongapo and Angeles. Six of the women have since become pregnant and at least three are known to have delivered.

Public concern that AIDS was being introduced to the Philippines by US servicemen led to protests and to calls to close the bases, particularly from a women's group, Gabriela. Regulations introduced in February 1988 mean that all foreign seamen will have to carry a Philippines-issued "AIDS Clearance Certificate" and that the US government guarantees all its military personnel have tested negative for HIV. A study of "sexually promiscuous" individuals showed 16% of men and 47% of women had had foreign partners. Anal intercourse was admitted to by almost half the men, but only 17% admitted taking the receptor role. The study also revealed heavy alcohol and drug intake and "rare use of condoms". Dr Thelma Tupasi, who led the study, warned of the "explosive potential" for the spread of AIDS [M.L.Tan, *Report on First International Conference on AIDS in Asia*, November 1987]. Ministry of health support for AIDS education programmes aimed at hospitality workers includes efforts to assist these workers in finding alternative employment.

SINGAPORE
First reported case: September 1986
Cases reported by January 1988: 4 (2 per million)
Seropositivity: To June 1987: 0/84 haemophiliacs, 3/107,833 (0.003%) blood donors, 9/183 (4.9%) homosexual/bisexual men, 0/2,466 prostitutes, 0/222, 2 others [CP].
Action: AIDS Advisory Committee set up and education campaign began in 1985.

Transfusion blood and donor semen for in vitro fertilisation screened.

SRI LANKA
First reported case: 1986
Cases reported by January 1988: 4 (0.1 per million). 2 Sri Lankans, 2 foreign.
Seropositivity: To January 1988: 0/20,000 of individuals at high risk tested HIV+ [HMC].
Action: MTP from June 1988, TSA from December 1987.

The first registered case was a British homosexual who was expelled in November 1987.

THAILAND
First diagnosed case: 1984
Cases reported by December 1987: 12 (0.2 per million). All male, all homosexual; 4 foreign, 8 Thai.
Seropositivity: To October 1987: 69/2,656 (2.6%) male sex workers, 7/12,873 (0.05%) female sex workers, 6/44,741 (0.01%) blood donors, 78/15,877 (0.5%) prisoners, 6/711 (0.8%) drug addicts [*Nation*, Bangkok, 6 December 1987]. December 1987: total of 27 ARC cases and 158 cases of HIV-positivity identified [HMC]. March 1988: 15% of 1,600 ivdus (compared with 1% in March 1987) [*Le Monde*, Paris, 7 April 1987].
Action: MTP from July 1988.
Entry restrictions: People with AIDS.

In August 1987 a national AIDS campaign was launched with a four year budget of 43m baht (US$1.7m); 20m baht was scheduled to be spent on research. In the same year 170m baht (US$6.7m) was spent overseas promoting tourism. [*Nation*, Bangkok, 13 September 1987]. Organisations within Thailand have alleged that the anti-AIDS campaign has a low profile because it might discourage tourism, the country's primary source of foreign currency. The high percentage of HIV+ drug users detected in early 1988 suggests imminent entry of the virus into this population (see Chapter Four).

VIETNAM
No cases of AIDS reported by May 1988.
Seropositivity: 1987: 0/1,000 "high-risk group" members (prostitutes, drug addicts, STD patients) [HMC].
Action: Assessment visit.

The government intends to screen 100,000 individuals throughout the country in the next three years [HMC].

....

OCEANIA

REPORTED AIDS CASES at June 1988

	Officially reported Aids cases	Population (in millions)	AIDS cases per million population
Australia	872	16.20	54
New Zealand	84	3.30	25

These figures exclude countries reporting fewer than 10 cases. Sourece: Panos, from WHO and nationa health ministry figures.

Most countries in the region are less-developed island states or territories heavily dependent on natural resource exports, tourism or, in the case of the smallest islands, grants from sympathetic governments. Apart from Australia and New Zealand, where AIDS appeared several years ago, mostly in homosexual men, no cases were diagnosed in Oceania until 1987. The main source of infection appears to be tourists and islanders returning from working abroad. Intravenous drug abuse in the region is uncommon and in the larger islands at least screening of blood donations is now in operation.

Reminder: Seropositivity studies of a specific segment of a population (eg prostitutes or blood donors in a large city) should *not* be taken as representative of the country as a whole.

AUSTRALIA
First reported case: 1982
Cases reported April 1988: 872   (54 per million.
Breakdown: At 30 July 1987: 86.5% homosexual contact, 7.8% blood product recipients. 3.0% homosexual/ivdu, 1.6% heterosexual contact, 0.5% ivdu, 0.5% undetermined; 95.9% male, 4.1% female.
Seropositivity: April 1987: 50,000 (0.3% of population) estimated HIV+ [*Independent*, London 6 April 1987].
Action: National Advisory Committee on AIDS set up in November 1984; its budget for 1986-87 was A$11.6 million.

Although homosexual activity was the primary means of transmission amongst diagnosed cases, one report suggested that 172,000 Australians were at least casual intravenous drug users, equivalent to almost 1 in 100 of the population; equally worrying was the report that needles were shared by 60% of drug users [*Independent*, London, 6 April 1987].

National education campaign launched in early 1987 with a budget of A$3 million (US$2,100,000), and featured a television commercial with Death in a bowling alley knocking down human bowling-pins. To reach the large immigrant population, leaflets were prepared in 16 languages, radio advertisements in 58 languages and the television commercial in 11 languages. A campaign directed at the indigenous population involving Aborigines in design and planning from the beginning has been seen as a model for campaigns directed at minority populations elsewhere. Three months after the campaign was launched surveys revealed a significant increase in knowledge and increased condom use [*Nacaids Campaign Three Months On;* paper published by the National Advisory Committee on AIDS, 1987]. Transfusion blood screened since April 1985.

FIJI

No AIDS cases reported or epidemiological studies published by March 1988. Government education campaign began in 1985 in English and Fijian, utilising radio, newspapers, brochures and posters; also special campaign directed at homosexuals [CP].

FRENCH POLYNESIA (Overseas Département of France)
First reported case: 1987
Cases reported January 1988: : 1 (5 per million)
Seropositivity: To January 1987: 1/138 (0.7%) homosexual men, 9/170 (5.3%) homo/bisexual men and 1/74 (1.3%) women attending private doctors or STD clinics, 6/125 (4.8%) blood product recipients; in addition a sexual partner of one of the above tested positive [E. Chungue et al, WICA, p 78]. Mid-1987: 30/16,000 (0.2%) blood donors and people at high risk [CP].
Action: Territorial AIDS Commission set up February 1986.

Almost all who tested positive had contracted the virus abroad. One homosexual man who had never left French Polynesia had a number of foreign partners. Education campaign in French and Tahitian began in 1986; all forms of the media were utilised. Education in schools scheduled to begin toward the end of 1987 [CP].

NEW ZEALAND
First reported case: 1984
Cases reported April 1988: 84 (25 per million)
Transfusion blood is screened.

PAPUA NEW GUINEA
No AIDS cases reported to WHO by March 1988.
Seropositivity: To February 1988: 4/1,000 (0.004%) HIV+ (2 homosexuals, 2 female nationals) [draft proposal for an AIDS prevention and control programme in Papua New Guinea, February 1988].
Entry restrictions: work permit applicants.
Transfusion blood is partially screened.

TONGA
First reported case: 1987
Cases reported October 1987: 1 (10 per million)
VANUATU
No AIDS cases reported by June 1988.
Seropositivity: 1986: 0/102 random samples [CP].
Education campaign scheduled to begin in early 1988.

No other island in the region has reported cases of AIDS or has published epidemiological studies, so far as Panos is aware.

NO AIDS TEST, NO ENTRY

The number of countries imposing AIDS-related restrictions has more than doubled in the year to mid-1988. These countries believe that the best way of preventing the epidemic from spreading is to stop all those who might be carrying the virus from entering their country. So far, however, the World Health Organization's advice against screening tourists has been generally accepted.

The blood test, which is often — and erroneously — referred to as an "AIDS test" is not really a test for AIDS. It is a test which shows whether a person has produced antibodies in response to HIV, the virus which causes AIDS. Where testing for HIV is a requirement, a positive result almost always means deportation or refusal to issue the relevant visa.

There are two problems associated with the test. Because it takes several months, and sometimes longer than a year, before the test registers exposure to the virus, recently-exposed people may test negative even though they are not. On the other hand, a very small percentage of people test positive even though they have had no contact with HIV.

Most countries demanding the test expect it to be carried out in the traveller's country of origin. This makes the impact of such regulations difficult to gauge. Panos has no way of knowing how many people change their plans because of a positive result.

In researching travel restrictions and AIDS, Panos has often come across conflicting information. One branch of government may not inform another when announcing new restrictions. Different levels of government may disagree over new regulations. The government may not inform its embassies abroad. The decision may be taken in secret and not announced at all. Testing may be officially announced and then withdrawn or "forgotten". What follows is a summary of the information available to Panos on 1 July 1988.

BELGIUM: Foreign students receiving a scholarship from the Ministry of Foreign Affairs, Foreign Trade and Development Co-operation must take an HIV-antibody test in their country of origin.

BELIZE: Applicants for naturalisation, work or residence permits must take an HIV-antibody test.

BULGARIA: All foreigners staying longer than one month and all Bulgarians returning from working abroad must take an HIV-antibody test within three days of arrival. Students testing positive are known to have been deported.

CHINA: All foreigners staying longer than one year must take an HIV-antibody test. Visitors staying for less time are not tested, but those discovered to be carrying the virus have been placed in isolation and deported.

COSTA RICA: Foreign students and all applicants for residence must take an HIV-antibody test.

CUBA: Foreigners (but not tourists) and Cubans returning from "endemic areas" must take an HIV-antibody test. If negative, the test is repeated six months later.

CYPRUS: Foreigners seeking work permits to work in nightclubs or as cabaret artists and all students from African countries must take an HIV-antibody test.

CZECHOSLOVAKIA: Foreign students must take an HIV-antibody test; Some HIV-positives have been deported.

EGYPT: Foreign defence contractors working at military establishments must "carry an HIV-antibody test certificate".

FINLAND: There are conflicting reports as to whether foreign students must take an HIV-antibody test.

FEDERAL REPUBLIC OF GERMANY (WEST GERMANY): All students receiving a scholarship from the Ministry of Economic Co-operation must take an HIV-antibody test in their country of origin. Visas granted in certain African countries may be invalidated on "health grounds". In the state of Bavaria, all foreigners applying for a residence permit must take an HIV-antibody test; nationals of the European Community and all other western European countries are excepted.

INDIA: All foreign students must take an HIV-antibody test. Students testing positive are known to have been deported.

INDONESIA: Foreigners with AIDS may not enter the country, but visitors are not generally required to take an HIV- antibody test.

IRAQ: All foreigners staying longer than five days and all Iraqis returning from abroad must take an HIV-antibody test.

ISRAEL: Press reports indicate that restrictions on some or all foreign visitors are being considered.

JAMAICA: Press reports indicate that restrictions on some or all foreign visitors are being considered.

JAPAN: Press reports indicate that restrictions on some or all foreign visitors are being considered.

REPUBLIC OF KOREA (SOUTH KOREA): Press reports indicate that restrictions on some or all foreign visitors may be introduced after the 1988 Olympics.

KUWAIT: Residence and work permit applicants must take an HIV- antibody test.

LIBYA: Foreign students and applicants for "residence for professional purposes" must carry an "AIDS certificate".

MONGOLIA: Foreign students must take an HIV-antibody test on arrival, to be repeated "several months" later.

PAPUA NEW GUINEA: Work permits will only be issued upon presentation of a valid "AIDS certificate".

PHILIPPINES: HIV-antibody tests are required for applicants for permanent visas and, reportedly, for foreign seaman.

POLAND: Foreign students must take an HIV-antibody test either in their country of origin or on arrival.

QATAR: Residence and work permit applicants must present an "AIDS certificate" issued within the preceding six months.

SAUDI ARABIA: Foreigners seeking a work permit for longer than one month must take an HIV-antibody test in their country of origin at a hospital recognised by the Saudi authorities.

SOUTH AFRICA: All foreigners (as well as citizens) may be required to take an HIV-antibody test on demand, but press reports indicate this measure is only being applied to foreign black applicants for work permits.

SOVIET UNION: Foreigners staying longer than three months must take an HIV-antibody test. Students testing positive are known to have been deported.

SRI LANKA: A Briton with AIDS is known to have been deported.

SYRIA: Students and work permit applicants must take an HIV- antibody test on arrival.

THAILAND: Foreigners with AIDS may not enter the country, but no test is required.

UNITED ARAB EMIRATES: Applicants for work permits must take an HIV-antibody test.

UNITED STATES: All applicants for immigrant visas must take an HIV-antibody test, in their country of origin unless they are already in the United States.

PEOPLE'S DEMOCRATIC REPUBLIC OF YEMEN (SOUTH YEMEN): Press reports indicate that foreigners testing positive for HIV antibodies have been deported.

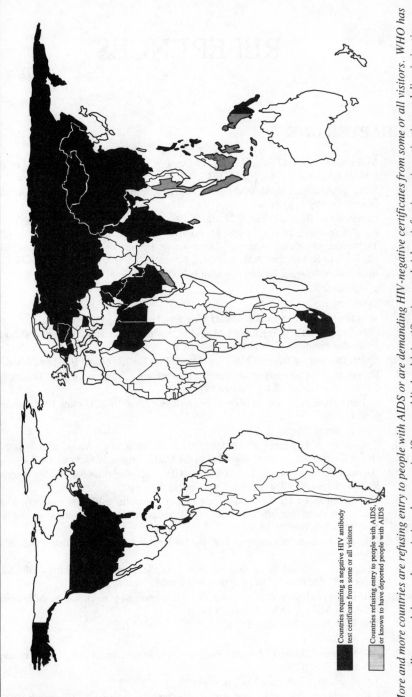

More and more countries are refusing entry to people with AIDS or are demanding HIV-negative certificates from some or all visitors. WHO has repeatedly argued that such restrictions have no significant public health justification, and risk reinforcing stigmatisation and discrimination against people infected with the virus. . Source: Panos

Countries requiring a negative HIV antibody test certificate from some or all visitors

Countries refusing entry to people with AIDS, or known to have deported people with AIDS

REFERENCES

CHAPTER ONE

1. M. Popovic and S. Gartner, *Lancet*, 17 October 1987, p916; and J. Nelson et al, *Lancet*, 6 February 1988, pp259-262.
2. M. L. Schiattone et al, *Abstracts of the Fourth International Conference on AIDS*, Stockholm, 1988, p171.
3. *International Herald Tribune*, 24 March 1988.
4. *Le Monde*, Paris, 24 April 1988; M. Popovic and S. Gartner, as reference 1; E. Tschachler et al, *Journal of Investigative Dermatology*, 1987, volume 88, p233-37; L. R. Braathen et al, *Lancet*, 7 November 1987, p1,094.
5. *International Herald Tribune*, 24 March 1988.
6. as reference 5.
7. as reference 5.
8. as reference 5, quoting Dr Daniel Bolgnesi, Duke University.
9. "Confronting AIDS", Insitute of Medicine, National Academy of Sciences, June 1988, Washington DC: National Academy Press.
10. I. Grant, *Annals of Internal Medicine*, December 1987, volume 107, pp828-836.
11. Report of the Consultation on the Neuropsychiatric Aspects of HIV Infection, GPA/WHO, Geneva, 14-17 March 1988.
12. H. Farzadegan et al, *Annals of Internal Medicine*, June 1988, volume 108, number 6, pp785-90.
13. New Scientist, 26 may 1988, p40.
14. Testimony of Lawrence Miike, US Office of Technology Assessment, to the House Committee on Small Business of the US Congress, 19 October 1987.
15. "Update: Serologic testing for antibody to HIV", *Morbidity and Mortality Weekly Review*, 8 January 1988, volume 36, number 52, pp1-8.
16. The British approach, based on the use of the competitive ELISA antibody test, and the reasons for its adoption are discussed in: R. Tedder, *Bulletin Institut Pasteur*, 1986, volume 84, pp405-413.
17. Office of Assistant Secretary of Defense for Health Affairs, Washington DC, July 1988.
18. Programme national de la lutte contre le SIDA: plan moyen terme, 1988-92, provisional document, Zaire department of public health, 93pp.
19. G. Slutkin et al, presentation to the First International Conference on the Global Impact of AIDS, London, March 1988.
20. *New York Times*, 2 January 1988.
21. as reference 20.
22. J.M. Mann et al, *Journal of the American Medical Association*, 18 July 1986, volume 256, number 3, p346.
23. *New Scientist*, 4 February 1988, p34.
24. L.B. Reichman, *Journal of the American Medical* Association, 12 December 1986, volume 256, number 22, p3,093.

25. *New Scientist*, 4 February 1988, p34.
26. Personal communication, Dr Richard Tedder, October 1986.
27. See for example Larry Kramer, *The Normal Heart*, New York City, 1985; Randy Shilts, *And the Band Played On*, 1987, St Martin's Press, New York, 630pp.
28. Address to American Foundation for AIDS Research fundraising dinner, June 1987, Washington DC.
29. Quotes from interview with Richard Rector published in *Blaming Others: Prejudice, race and worldwide AIDS*, Panos, London and Washington DC, 176pp.

CHAPTER TWO

1. A.R. Moss et al, *British Medical Journal*, 12 March 1988, pp745-50.
2. *USA Today*, 15 March 1988.
3. N. A. Hessol et al, Abstracts of the 3rd International Conference on AIDS, Washington DC, 1987, p1.
4. H.R. Brodt et al, *Deutsche Medizinische Wochenscrift*, 1985, volume 111, pp1,175-80.
5. Testimony by Dr Anthony Fauci to the President's AIDS committee, quoted in the *New York Times*, 15 February 1988.
6. Interview with Dr Anthony Fauci, December 1987.
7 Interview with Dr Richard Tedder, September 1987.
8. "Confronting AIDS", Institute of Medicine, National Academy of the Sciences, National Academy Press, Washington DC, June 1988.
9. Interviews with Dr Robert Gallo (June 1987) and Dr Richard Tedder (September 1987).
10. Interview with Dr Robert Gallo (June 1987).
11. Report of an oral presentation by Dr Francoise Barre-Sinoussi, *New Scientist*, 26 May 1988, p41.
12. Explanation of the hypotheses of Drs R. F. Cathcart and Russ Jaffe in M. A. Weiner, *Maximum Immunity*, Gateway Books, Bath, UK, 1986.
13. R. Rothenberg et al, *New England Journal of Medicine*, 19 November 1987, volume 317, number 21, pp1,297-1,302.
14. *Sunday Times*, London, 10 April 1988.
15. as reference 13.
16. New York Commission on Human Rights, "AIDS and people of color: the discriminatory impact," updated report, August 1987.
17. *Washington Post*, 1 October 1987.
18. D. Campbell, "The Amazing AIDS Scam", *New Statesman and Society*, 24 June 1988.
19. *New England Journal of Medicine*, Special Report, 26 February 1987, volume 316, number 9 pp557-64.
20. *New Scientist*, 17 March 1988, p30.
21. Information presented verbally to a workshop on AZT at the Fourth International Conference on AIDS, Stockholm, 12-16 June 1988.
22. *Washington Post*, 25 February 1988.
23. *Toronto Globe and Mail*, 1 March 1988.
24. *USA Today*, 3 September 1987.

25. as reference 18.
26. M. J. Wood and A. M. Geddes, *Lancet*, July 1987, pp1189-1193.
27. *New York Times*, 18 December 1987.
28. *New Scientist*, 21 April 1988, p21.
29. *New York Times*, 16 February 1988.
30. Dr Jerome Groopman, quoted in the *New York Times*, 16 February 1988.
31. *International Herald Tribune*, 30 August 1987 and *New York Times*, 16 February 1988.
32. *Times*, London, 25 April 1988.
33. P. L. Nara et al, Abstracts of the Fourth International Conference on AIDS, June 1988, p146.
34. *New York Times*, 12 February 1988.
35. D. M. Barnes, *Science*, 5 September 1986, volume 233, p1,035.

CHAPTER THREE

1. R. J. Biggar et al (edit.), *European Journal of Cancer and Clinical Oncology*, 1984, volume 20, number 2, pp157-73; N. Clumeck et al, *Lancet*, 19 March 1983, p642; J.B. Brunet and R.A. Ancelle, *Annals of Internal Medicine*, November 1985, volume 103, number 5, pp670-4.
2. A.M. Hardy et al, *Public Health Report*, July/August 1987, volume 102, pp386-91.
3. Interview with Dr Jonathan Mann, head of Global Programme on AIDS, World Health Organization, April 1988.
4. Interview with Dr Ron St John, Co-ordinator, Health Situation and Trend Assessment Program, Pan American Health Organization, January 1988.
5. P. Piot et al, *Science*, 5 February 1988, volume 239, pp573- 579.
6. as reference 5.
7. J. M. Mann, statement given in an informal briefing to the 42nd session of the United Nations General Assembly, 20 October 1987.
8. A. M. Hardy et al, *Journal of the American Medical Association*, volume 253, number 22, 11 January 1985, pp215-220.
9. *Global WHO Strategy for the Prevention and Control of Acquired Immunodeficiency Syndrome: Projected Needs for 1986-87*, WHO Geneva, 1986.
10. UNICEF, *The State of the World's Children 1988*, Oxford University Press.
11. Speech by J.M. Mann at World Health Ministers Conference, London, January 1988.
12. F. Clavel et al, *Science*, volume 233, 18 July 1986, pp343-346.
13. A. Outtara et al, *Annals de l'Institut Pasteur/Virologie*, August 1986, 137E, pp303-10.
14. A. G. Saimot et al & R. Ancelle et al, *Lancet*, 21 March 1987, pp688-9.
15. L. Sangare et al, *Abstracts of the Second International Symposium on AIDS and Associated Cancers in Africa*, Naples, 1987, p81.
16. R.C. Kooiman et al, Abstracts of the First Conference on the Global Impact of AIDS, London, March 1988, p26.
17. F. Schon and J.Blau, *Lancet*, 23 January 1988, pp188-9.
18. D. C. W. Mabey et al, *British Medical Journal*, 9 January 1988, volume 286, pp83-6.
19. K. Kourouma et al, *Abstracts of the Second International Symposium on AIDS and*

Associated Cancers in Africa, Naples, 1987, pp79-80.

20.　J. M. Allaire et al, *Abstracts of the Third International Conference on* AIDS, Washington DC, 1987, p23.

21.　Presentation by delegate at Health Ministers' Conference, London, January 1988.

22.　as reference 14.

23.　C. Krögel et al, *Lancet*, 16 May 1987.

24.　*Global Disease Surveillance Report*, August 1987.

25.　*Guardian*, London, 21 March 1988.

26.　*New Scientist*, 20 August 1987.

27.　*Morbidity and Mortality Weekly Report*, 29 January 1988.

28.　R.V. Henrickson et al, *Lancet*, 19 February 1983, pp388-90.

29.　M. D. Daniel et al, *Papers from Science, 1982-1985*, Washington: The American Association for the Advancement of Science, pp484-489; P. J. Kanki et al, *Papers from Science, 1982-1985*, pp490-495.

30.　H. Kornfeld et al, *Nature*, 9 April 1987, volume 326, pp610- 13.

31.　*Nature*, 18 February 1988, volume 331, p621.

32.　*Nature*, 2 June 1988, volume 333, p396.

33.　T. F. Smith et al, *Nature*, 9 June 1988, volume 333, p494.

34.　as reference 31.

35.　*Nature*, 9 June 1988, volume 333, p494.

36.　as reference 5.

37.　*Weekly Epidemiological Record*, 8 April 1988, pp105-107.

38.　J. W. Pape et al, *Clinical Research*, volume 34, number 2, 1986, p528.

39.　A presentation by J. Hospedales at the First Conference on the Global Impact of AIDS, March 1988.

40.　See for example R. Parker, *Medical Anthropology Quarterly,* new series, volume 1, number 2, June 1987, pp155-175; J. M. Carrier, Archives of Sexual Behaviour, volume 5, number 2, 1976, pp103-124.

41.　*Le Monde*, Paris, 24 June 1987.

42.　Concepts of heterosexuality and homosexuality are relatively new in Latin America and men tend to identify themselves as to whether they take the active or passive role in intercourse. See papers in reference 40.

43.　*International Herald Tribune*, 15 February 1988.

44.　as reference 43.

45.　A. J. France et al, *British Medical Journal*, 20 February 1988, volume 296, pp526-9.

46.　T. C. Quinn et al, *New England Journal of Medicine*, 28 January 1988, pp197-203.

47.　R. M. Anderson and R. M. May, *Nature,* 9 June 1988, volume 333, pp514-9.

CHAPTER FOUR

1.　New York City Department of Public Health, news release "Number of newly reported AIDS cases in IV drug users eclipses number of cases in gay and bisexual men", 16 April 1988.

2.　J.W. Curran et al, *Science*, 5 February 1988, volume 239, pp610-6.

3.　Interview with Don Edwards, Executive Director, US National Minority AIDS

Council, June 1988; interview with Dr David Walters, Director, Canadian Public Health Association, June 1988.

4. as reference 2.

5. D.R. Hopkins, address to National Conference on AIDS in Minority Populations in the United States, Atlanta, 8 August 1987.

6. *Morbidity and Mortality Weekly Report*, 15 May 1987, volume 36, number 18, pp273-6.

7. P. Piot et al, *Science*, 5 February 1988, volume 239, pp573- 579; from the *Abstracts of the Third International Conference on AIDS*, Washington DC, 1987: M. Braddick et al, p158: N. Nzila et al, p158: H. Francis et al, p214; from the *Abstracts of the Second International Conference on AIDS in Africa*, Naples, 1987: W. Nsa et al, p121; J. K. Kreiss et al, p64: E. Baende et al, p121; F. Denis et al, *Lancet*, 1987-I, 408.

8. P. Piot et al, as reference 7; R. Ancelle-Park et al, *Lancet*, 1987, number 2, p626; J.B. Brunet et al, *AIDS*, 1, 59 (1987).

9. P. Piot et al, as reference 7, including papers mentioned in article.

10. as reference 7.

11. Unpublished study by New York City Department of Public Health.

12. *Independent*, London, 14 January 1988.

13. P. Piot et al, *Abstracts of the Second International Conference on AIDS*, Paris, June 1986, p101.

14. S. Landesman et al, *Journal of the American Medical Association*, November 20 1987, volume 258, number 19, pp2701- 3.

15. R. Hoff et al, *New England Journal of Medicine*, 3 March 1988, volume 318, number 9, pp525-30.

16. *Washington Post*, 10 October 1987.

17. Report on the Ministry of Health Seminar on AIDS, 24-26 July 1986, University Teaching Hospital, Lusaka, unpublished, 5pp.

18. G. B. Scott et al, *Journal of the American Medical Association*, 1985, volume 253, pp363-366.

19. For a recent example see Randy Shilts, *And the Band Played On*, New York, St Martin's Press, 1987, pp630.

20. R. M. May, *Nature*, 25 February 1988, volume 331, pp655-6.

21. P. Piot et al, as reference 7.

22. H. Handsfield et al, Abstracts of the Third International Conference on AIDS, Washington DC, June 1987, p206; J.W. Curran et al, *Science*, 5 February 1988, volume 239, pp610-6; J. Kreiss et al, *Genitourinary Medicine*, 1988, volume 64, pp1-2.

23. P. Piot et al, as reference 7.

24. W. Winkelstein et al, *Journal of the American Medical* Association, 16 January 1987, volume 257, number 3, pp321-5; J. Levy et al, *Lancet*, 6 February 1988, pp259-62.

25. R. J. Pomerantz et al, *Annals of Internal Medicine*, March 1988, volume 108, pp321-7.

26. P. Piot et al, as reference 7.

27. F. Plummer et al, *Abstracts of the Third International Conference on AIDS*, Washington DC, June 1987, p6.

28. A. S. Latif et al, *Abstracts of the African Regional Conference on Sexually Transmitted Diseases*, Harare, Zimbabwe, June 1987, p7.

29. D. W. Cameron et al, *Abstracts of the Fourth International Conference on AIDS*,

12-Stockholm, 16 June 1988, p275.

30. Dr Francis Plummer, interview, Fourth International Conference on AIDS, Stockholm, 12-16 June 1988.

31. Dr Allan Ronald, comments during presentation to the Fourth International Conference on AIDS, Stockholm, 12-16 June 1988.

32. P. Piot et al, as reference 7; Cameron et al, *Abstracts of the Third International Conference on AIDS*, Washington DC, 1987, p25.

33. J.K. Kreiss et al, *Annals of Internal Medicine*, May 1985, volume 102, number 5, pp623-626; J.M. Jason et al, *Journal of the American Medical* Association, 10 January 1986, volume 255, pp212-215; *Morbidity and Mortality Weekly Report*, 11 September 1987, number 36, p593; T. A. Peterman et al, *Abstracts of the Second International Conference on AIDS*, Paris, 1986, p107.

34. O. P. Arya and J. B. Lawson, *Tropical Doctor*, April 1977, volume 7, pp51-6.

35. P. Piot and A. Meheus, *Annals de la Socit Belge de Médecine Tropicale*, 1983, volume 63, pp87-110.

36. A.O Osoba, *British Journal of Venereal Diseases*, 1981, volume 57, pp89-94.

37. as reference 36.

38. as reference 36.

39. as reference 34.

40. *Weekly Epidemiological Record*, 8 April 1988.

41. *Weekly Epidemiological Record*, 10 January 1986.

42. *Independent*, London, 6 April 1987.

43. See reference to the need to struggle against "defeatism" in the foreword by WHO director-general Dr Halfdan Mahler to *Progress Report Number 2: November 1987*, Special Programme on AIDS, WHO/SPA/Geneva/87.4.

44. R. M. Anderson et al, *Nature*, volume 332, pp228-234.

45. as reference 44, p231.

46. See for example J.C. Cutler and R.C. Arnold, *American Journal of Public Health*, April 1988, volume 78, number 4, pp372-6.

47. E. Drucker, *American Journal of Drug and Alcohol Abuse*, 12(1 & 2), 1986, pp165-181.

48. R.E. Chaisson et al, *American Journal of Public Health*, February 1987, 77(2) pp169-172.

49. A. M. Brandt, *American Journal of Public Health*, April 1988, volume 78, number 4, pp367-71.

50. *Washington Post*, 21 March 1988.

51. N. Nzilambi et al, *New England Journal of Medicine*, 4 February 1988, volume 318, number 5, pp276-9.

CHAPTER FIVE

1. *Population Reports*, Series 11, number 6, September-October 1982.

2. as reference 1.

3. For example see P. Van de Peree et al, *AIDS*, 1987, volume 1, number 1, 49-51.

4. J.M. Mann et al, *New England Journal of Medicine*, 15 February 1987, volume 36, number 6, p345.

5. M.A. Fischl et al, *Abstracts of the Third International Conference on AIDS*, Washington, 1987, p178.

6. *New Scientist*, 7 January 1988.

7. *Independent*, London, 19 June 1987.

8. *USA Today*, 12 February 1988.

9. *Lancet*, 21 November 1987, p1,224.

10. *Newsweek*, 8 February 1988.

11. Information from Sarita Kumar, International Planned Parenthood Federation, New York, May 1988.

12. as reference 11.

13. *AIDS Watch*, number 1, January 1988.

14. Information from Malc Okunnu, International Planned Parenthood Federation, London, May 1988.

15. *Independent*, London, 21 April 1988.

16. In recent years the Terrence Higgins Trust has expanded its base to include all sections of the community.

17. P. S. Arno, *Abstracts of the Second International Conference on AIDS*, Paris, 1986, p176.

18. *Guardian*, London, 18 February 1988; *Independent*, London, 25 March 1988.

19. Article written by the Tokyo correspondent London *Guardian* for the Panos book *Blaming Others*, July 1987.

20. Interview with Sunny Rumsey, New York City Department of Health, November 1987.

21. Interview with Don Edwards, National Minority AIDS Council, November 1987.

22. Excerpt from contribution by Dave Moyo in Panos book *Blaming Others*, July 1987.

23. *Monthly Life*, Lagos, May 1987.

24. Interview with Chris Jacques, New York City Department of Health, September 1987.

25. *International Herald Tribune*, 26 March 1988.

26. Interview with Dr June Osborne, June 1988.

27. Richard Parker, presentation at the annual conference of the American Association for the Advancement of Science, Boston, USA, February 1988.

28. Interview with Dr Ron St John, Pan American Health Organization, January 1988.

29. Article by Lazaro Timmo, Tanzanian journalist, for Panos book *Blaming Others*, July 1987.

30. V. M. Mays and S. D. Cochrane, *Public Health Reports*, March- April 1987, volume 102, number 2, pp224-31.

31. as reference 30.

32. Article by Zambian journalist Dave Moyo, written for the Panos Feature Service, 10 April 1987.

33. *Washington Post*, 28 December 1987.

34. *International Herald Tribune*, 1 October 1987.

35. as reference 29.

36. *International Herald Tribune*, 26 March 1988.

37. A. M. Brandt, *American Journal of Public Health*, April 1988, volume 78, number 4, pp367-371.

38. *New York Times*, 28 February 1988.

39. *Guardian*, London, 8 March 1988.
40. Interview with Dr Daniel Tarantola, National Programmes Support, WHO, June 1988.
41. S. Allen et al, *Abstracts of the Fourth International Conference on AIDS*, Stockholm, 1988, volume1, p349.
42. as reference 40. Support, WHO, June 1988.
43. *Herald*, Harare, 11 September 1987.
44. *New Scientist*, 12 May 1988.
45. as reference 40.
46. *New African*, London, July 1987.
47. *New York Times*, 4 June, 1988.
48. *African Concord*, Lagos, 5 April 1988.
49. P. Piot et al, *Science*, 5 February 1988, volume 239, pp573-86.
50. "Reaching the hard to reach", paper by E.N. Ngugi at the Health Ministers Conference, London, January 1988.
51. Personal communication, Brenda Stolzfus, May 1987.
52. Thai Ministry of Health statistics quoted in the *Nation*, Bangkok, 6 December 1987.
53. Interview with David Cueny, November 1987.
54. as reference 53.
55. Interview with Arturo Olivas, June 1988.
56. Based on information from market research survey carried out by Profamilia, the Family Planning Association of the Dominican Republic, 1987.
57. Dr Ruhakana Rugunda, speaking at the AMFAR-Panos Consultation on AIDS and Development, Talloires, France, March 1987.

CHAPTER SIX

1. R. W. Smith, "The National Impact of Negativistic Leadership", Presented at the 1987 Meeting of the Western Political Sciences Association, Anaheim, 26-28 March 1987.
2. Dr Jonathan Mann, director, Global Programme on AIDS, WHO; statement to the UN General Assembly, New York, 20 October 1987.
3. *Morbidity and Mortality Weekly Report*, 9 July 1982, volume 31, number 26, pp353-361.
4. *New York Times*, 3 July 1983.
5. Personal communication, Dr Jean Pape, October 1987.
6. *Morbidity and Mortality Weekly Report*, 10 May 1985, volume 34, number 18, pp245-248.
7. *AIDS and People of Color: the Discriminatory Impact*, the AIDS Discrimination Unit of the New York City Commission on Human Rights, August 1987, pp23-4.
8. *New York Times*, 29 November 1983 and 11 October 1984.
9. N. Clumeck et al, *Lancet*, 19 March 1983, p642; N. Clumeck et al, *New England Journal of Medicine*, 23 February 1984, volume 310, pp492-7; J. B. Brunet et al, *Lancet*, 26 March 1983, pp700-1.
10. R.J. Biggar et al, *International Journal of Cancer*, 15 June 1985, volume 35, pp763-7.

11. W. C. Saxinger et al, *Science,* 1 March 1985, volume 227, pp1,036-38.
12. *Los Angeles Times,* 22 February 1985.
13. as reference 10; D. Serwadda et al, *Lancet,* 19 October 1985, pp849-52.
14. R. Tedder, *Bulletin Institut Pasteur,* 1986, number 84, pp405-13.
15. For example see: J. A. Levy et al, *Proceedings of the National Academy of the Sciences,* October 1986, volume 83, number 20, pp7,935-7; S.F. Lyons et al, *New England Journal of Medicine,* 9 May 1985, volume 312, number 19, pp 1257-8; Anonymous, *AIDS Forschung,* January 1987, volume 1, pp5-25.
16. A. J.Nahnias et al, *Lancet,* 31 May 1986, pp1,279-80.
17. *Morbidity and Mortality Weekly Report,* 5 June 1981, volume 30, number 21, pp250-2; M. Gottlieb et al, *New England Journal of Medicine,* 10 December 1981, volume 305, number 24, pp1,425-1,431.
18. For a narrative account of the dawning awareness of a new immunodeficiency disease in the US see Randy Shilts, *And the Band Played On,* New York, St. Martin's Press, 1987, 630pp.
19. B. Lamey and N. Malemeka, *Médecine Tropicale,* September-October 1982, volume 42, number 5, pp507-11.
20. A C. Bayley, *Lancet,* 16 June 1984, pp1,318-20.
21. J.Vandepitte et al, *Lancet,* 23 April 1983, pp924-6.
22. G. Offenstadt et al, *New England Journal of Medicine,* 31 March 1983, volume 308, p775.
23. R. J. Biggar et al (edit), *European Journal of Cancer and Clinical Oncology,* 1984, volume 20, number 2, pp157-73; N. Clumeck et al, *Lancet,* 19 March 1983, p642; J.B. Brunet and R. A. Ancelle, *Annals of Internal Medicine,* November 1985, volume 103, number 5, pp670-4.
24. J.W. Pape et al, *New England Journal of Medicine,* 20 October 1983, volume 309, number 16, pp945-50.
25. *Morbidity and Mortality Weekly Report,* 9 July 1982, volume 31, number 26, pp353-361.
26. *Chicago Tribune,* 25 October 1987.
27. T. Jonckheer et al. *Lancet,* 16 February 1985, pp400-1.
28. as reference 21.
29. C. Bygbjerg, *Lancet,* 23 April 1983, pp925.
30. S. S. Frøland et al, *Lancet,* 11 June 1988, pp1,344-5.
31. as reference 26.
32. as reference 26.
33. G. Williams et al, *Lancet,* 29 October 1960, pp951-955.
34. G. R. Hennigar et al, *American Journal of Clinical Pathology,* April 1961, volume 35, number 4, pp353-64.
35. *Economist,* London, 21 March 1987, p59; *Le Monde,* Paris, 27 July 1987.
36. *World Military and Social Expenditures,* Washington DC, 1985; *World Directory of Medical Schools,* WHO, 1979; *The World of Learning,* London, Europa Publications Ltd, 1986.
37. *La Gazette,* Yaoundé, 9 July 1987.
38. E. P. Assya, *Fraternité-Matin,* 8 August 1987 as quoted in J. Brooke, "In Cradle of AIDS Theory, a Defensive Africa Sees a Disguise for Racism", *New York Times,* 19 November 1987.
39. *New Vision,* Kampala, 10 February 1987.
40. *New York Times,* 19 November 1987.

41. *African Concord*, Lagos, 22 January 1987.
42. as reference 37.
43. *Standard*, Nairobi, 14 January 1987.
44. *Sunday Telegraph*, London, 21 September 1986.
45. *Times of Zambia*, Lusaka, 23 September 1986.
46. Information on Zambian tourist industry from Zambian journalist Dave Moyo.
47. From text of Zambian letter, 13 October 1987, written to a British researcher.
48. *Times of Zambia*, Lusaka, 29 August 1987.
49. *Newswatch*, Lagos, 30 March 1987.
50. Interview with James Brooke, November 1987.

CHAPTER SEVEN

1. J. M. Mann, "AIDS epidemiology, impact, prevention and control: the WHO perspective", statement read by Dr O. T. Christiansen to the German Marshall Fund of the United States Conference, West Berlin, 25- 27 June 1987.
2. Anonymous, *AIDS-Forschung*, January 1987, volume 1, pp 5-25; P. Piot et al, *Science*, 5 February 1988, volume 239, pp573-9.
3. J. M. Mann et al, *Journal of American Medicine*, 20 June 1986, volume 255, number 23, pp3,255-9.
4. J. W. Curran et al, *Science*, 5 February 1988, volume 239, pp610-6.
5. P. Piot et al, as reference 2.
6. Dr Leonardo Mata, interview, October 1987.
7. *Abstracts of the Second International Symposium on AIDS and Associated Cancers in Africa*, Naples, October 1987.
8. *Weekly Epidemiological Review*, 11 March 1988, pp73-76.
9. J. M. Mann, statement given in an informal briefing to the 42nd session of the United Nations General Assembly, 20 October 1987.
10. *Guardian*, London, 11 March 1988.
11. as reference 1.
12. R. M. Anderson, presentation to the First International Conference on the Global Impact of AIDS, London, March 1988.
13 A. A. Scitovsky, presentation to the First International Conference on the Global Impact of AIDS, London, March 1988.
14. P. Piot et al, as reference 2.
15. as reference 13.
16. L. G. M. Rodrigues, presentation at Global Impact of AIDS conference, op. cit.
17. C. Ruiz et al, *Abstracts of the First International Conference on the Global Impact of AIDS*, London, 1988, p41.
18. M. Over, presentation at the First International Conference on the Global Impact of AIDS, London, March 1988.
19. as reference 18.
20. C. Meyers, Presentation on the Social and Economic Impact of AIDS in Developing Countries, Third International Conference on AIDS, Washington DC, June 1987.
21. B. M. Nkowane, *Abstracts of the First International Conference on the Global Impact of AIDS*, London, March 1988, p35.

22. as reference 21.
23. F. Davichi et al, *Abstracts of the First International Conference on the Global Impact of AIDS*, London, March 1988, p38.
24. as reference 18.
25. Comments by Herbert Lister, chairman of Allstate Life Insurance Company, at a meeting of 125 US companies, quoted in *Journal of the American Medical Association*, 13 November 1987, volume 258, number 18, pp2,479-80.
26. as references 13 and 18.
27. Quoted in *South* magazine, London, December 1987.
28. *Sunday Telegraph*, London, 21 September 1986.
29. Information on Zambian tourist industry from Zambian journalist Dave Moyo.
30. *International Herald Tribune*, 23 November 1985.
31. *Daily Nation*, Nairobi, 26 November 1986; *Kenya Times*, Nairobi, 4 December 1986.
32. *New York Times*, 29 November 1983.
33. as reference 32.
34. *The Talloires Conclusions*, Panos, London, 1987.
35. Written report to Panos by Hickloch Ogola, February 1988.
36. *Yearbook of Tourism Statistics*, volume 1, World Tourism Organization, Madrid, 1986, p81.
37. *Nation*, Bangkok, 13 September 1987.
38. Thai Ministry of Health statistics quoted in the Nation, Bangkok, 6 December 1987.
39. as reference 36.
40. *Indonesian Observer*, 21 January 1988.
41. as reference 36.
42. *Sun*, Colombo, 30 January 1987.
43. *New Scientist*, London, 14 April 1988.
44. E.N. Ngugi, "Reaching the hard to reach", presentation at Health Ministers Conference, London, January 1988.
45. as reference 43; also Panos sources.
46. Andrew Graham-Yooll in *South*, London, May 1988.
47. as reference 35.
48. *Daily Telegraph*, London, 12 May 1988.
49. *Nation*, Bangkok, 13 September 1987.
50. *Independent*, London, 24 February 1988.
51. Source: World Health Organization.
52. Source: World Bank, 1986 & 1987.

CHAPTER EIGHT

1. Dr Halfdan Mahler, speech to the final plenary session of the Fourth International Conference on AIDS, Stockholm, June 1988.
2. *The Global Eliminiation of Smallpox*, final report of the Global Commission for the certification of smallpox eradication, World Health Organization, Geneva, 1980, p64.
3. Dr Jonathan Mann, director, Global Programme on AIDS, WHO, from speech to World Summit of Health Ministers, London, January 1988.

4. Panos interview with Dr. Daniel Tarantola, National Programmes Support, Global Programme on AIDS, WHO, Geneva, March 1988.

5. as reference 4.

6. as reference 4.

7. as reference 4.

8. as reference 4.

9. Dr Halfdan Mahler, speech to the United Nations General Assembly, New York, 20 October 1988.

10. as reference 4.

11. Interview with Dr Jonathan Mann, director, Global Programme on AIDS, WHO, Geneva, March 1988.

12. Interview with Dr James Chin, Surveillance Forcasting and Impact Assessment Unit, Global Programme on AIDS, WHO, Geneva, March 1988

13. as reference 11.

14. Interview with Dr Manuel Carballo, Social and Behavioural Research Unit, Global Programme on AIDS, WHO, Geneva, March 1988.

15. Interview with Dr Michael Caraël, consultant to Social and Behavioural Research Unit, Global Programme on AIDS, WHO, Geneva, March 1988.

16 WHO consultation with NGOs, February 1988.

17. as reference 11.

18. Dr Jonathan Mann, director, Global Programme on AIDS, WHO, from speech at the First International Conference on the Global Impact of AIDS, London, March 1988.

19. Interview with Dr Ron St John, Coordinator of Health Situation and Trends Assessment Program, PAHO, Washington DC, January 1988.

20. Panos interview with Dr Fernando Zacarias, Regional Advisor on AIDS and STDs for the health situation and trend assessment programme, PAHO, Washington DC, June 1988.

21. as reference 19.

22. as reference 20.

23. Statement from the consultation on breast-feeding/breastmilk and human immunodeficiency virus (HIV), GPA/WHO, Geneva, 23-25 June 1987.

24. *Report on WHO Consultation on HIV and Routine Childhood Immunization*, WHO, Geneva, 12-13 August 1987.

25. Statement from the Consultation on Prevention and Control of AIDS in Prisons, GPA/WHO, Geneva, 16-18 November 1987.

26. *Report of the Consultation on the Neuropsychiatric Aspects of HIV Infection*, GPA/WHO, 14-17 March 1988.

27. *Social Aspects of AIDS Prevention and Control Programmes*, GPA/WHO, 1 December 1987.

28. *Meeting on HIV Infection and Drug Injecting Intervention Strategies*, GPA/WHO, Geneva, 18-20 January 1988.

29. *Report of the Meeting on Criteria for HIV Screening Programmes*, GPA/WHO, 20-21 May 1987.

30. *Report of the Consultation on International Travel and HIV Infection*, GPA/WHO, Geneva, 2-3 March 1987.

31. *AIDS and the Newborn*, Report on WHO Consultation, WHO, Copenhagen, 9-10 April 1987.

CHAPTER NINE

1. Quoted in L. Mott, *Ciência e Cultura*, January 1987, volume 39, number 1, pp4-13.
2. *Newsweek*, 31 August 1987.
3. *La Prensa*, Washington DC, 1 September 1987.
4. *Time*, 14 September 1987.
5. *India Today*, 31 January 1987.
6. *New Scientist*, London, 14 April 1988.
7. *Anti-Gay Violence, Victimization and Defamation in 1987*, National Gay Task Force, Washington DC, June 1988.
8. *San Francisco Sentinel*, 15 May 1987.
9. Travestis are men who take hormones and/or surgical implants to develop breasts and live as women; they generally retain their male genitalia.
10. *Daily Telegraph*, London, 4 January 1988; further details confirmed by Panos, May 1988.
11. *Daily News*, London, 6 July 1987.
12. *Evening Standard*, London, 24 April 1987.
13. *Fritt Fram*, Oslo, June-July 1987.
14. *New York Times*, 23 April 1988.
15. Information from the Brazilian Inter-Disciplinary AIDS Association, May 1988.
16. *Times*, London, 25 September 1987.
17. *New York Times*, 7 February 1988.
18. *USA Today*, 15/17 August 1987.
19. *Daily Telegraph*, London, March 1987.
20. Interview with Eric Smith, Nova Scotia Task Force on AIDS, April 1988; *Chronicle Herald*, Halifax, Ma., 29 August 1987.
21. *Libération*, Paris, 16 February 1988.
22. *Daily Telegraph*, London, 30 November 1987.
23. *Le Monde*, Paris, 4 February & 5 February 1988.
24. *Independent*, London, 23 January 1988.
25. *Financial Times*, London, 27 February 1987; *Le Monde*, Paris, 4 February 1988; *International Herald Tribune*, 11 March 1988.
26. *New York Times*, 29 November 1987.
27. Interview with Wilson Carswell, Family Health International, June 1988.
28. *USA Today*, 3 February 1988.
29. M. Goldsmith, *Journal of the American Medical Association*, 1987, 258 (18), 2,479-80.
30. as reference 29.
31. *Acquired Immune Deficiency: AIDS in the Workplace*, Office of Personnel Management, Washington DC, March 1988.
32. *AIDS and Employment*, Department of Employment & Health and Safety Executive, London, 1986.
33. *Financial Times*, London, 27 February 1987.
34. *Times*, London, 25 July 1987; *Independent*, London, 21 December 1987.
35. *AIDS-Forschung*, 1987, 2 (9), pp521-9; *Occupational Health and Safety*, 1987, 56 (9), 12.
36. *Newsweek*, 27 July 1987.
37. R. Shilts, *And The Band Played On*, St Martin's Press, New York, 1987, pp374-5.

38. Royal College of Nursing spokesperson, June 1988.
39. British Medical Association, 3rd Statement on AIDS, December 1986.
40. *Journal of the American Medical Association*, March 1988, p1,360.
41. *Morbidity and Mortality Weekly Report*, 21 August 1987 (Supplement).
42. "Teaching Macho Researchers Some Respect", *Scientist*, 30 May 1988.
43. See for example R. N. Link et al, *American Journal of Public Health*, April 1988, volume 78 number 4, pp455-9.
44. *Daily Telegraph*, 2 June 1988.
45. *The Thunderbolt*, Marietta, no date, number 320.
46. J. Coombs, *The CDL Report*, Arabi, Louisiana, August 1987, issue 98.
47. *L'Action*, Nice, July/ August 1987, p18.
48. *Independent*, London, 2 May 1988.
49. *What Homosexuals Do*, leaflet published in 1987 by Family Research Institute Inc. Lincoln, Nebraska, 1987.
50. as reference 49.
51. *Economist*, London, 28 May 1988.
52. *Folha de São Paulo*, 22 January 1987.
53. T.W. Harding, *Lancet*, 28 November 1987, pp1260-4.
54. as reference 53.
55. *Libration*, Paris, 7-8 May 1988.
56. *Washington Post*, 1 December 1987.
57. *Independent*, London, 17 February 1987.
58. *Washington Post*, 1 December 1987.
59. *Globe and Mail*, Toronto, 29 October 1987.
60. as reference 53.
61. *Jornal do Brasil*, Rio de Janeiro, 30 January 1987.
62. *New York Times*, 21 January 1988.
63. *Le Monde*, Paris, 4 May 1987.
64. *New York Times*, 21 January 1988.
65. *Daily Telegraph*, London, 26 October 1987.
66. *New York Times*, 5 February 1988.
67. Interview with Sommatra Troy, March 1988.
68. *Folha de São Paulo*, 22 January 1987.
69. *Daily Telegraph*, London, 21 August 1987.
70. as reference 53.
71. *International Herald Tribune*, 17 September 1987.
72. Speech by Cuban delegate at World Health Ministers' Conference, London, January 1988.
73. *Le Monde*, Paris, 4 May 1988.
74. *Global Disease Surveillance Report*, August 1987; Panos source, May 1988.
75. Department of Social Affairs, Stockholm, spokesperson, April 1988.
76. Personal Communication, Pushpa Girimasi, Express News Agency, New Delhi, June 1988.
77. *Times*, London, 17 March 1988.
78. *Independent*, London, 11 January 1988.
79. *Financial Times*, London, 6 April 1988.
80. *Tabular Information on Legal Instruments Dealing with AIDS and HIV Infection*,

WHO document WHO/GPA/HLE/88.1, June 1988.

81. as reference 80.
82. MTI press release, Budapest, 10 June 1988.
83. as reference 80.
84. *Voice*, London, 9 February 1988.
85. *Times*, London, 11 January 1988.
86. *New Scientist*, 4 February 1988.
87. as reference 80.
88. as reference 80.
89. *Washington Post*, 26 April 1988.
90. *New York Times*, 29 April 1988; *New York Native*, 13 June 1988.
91. *New York Times*, 10 March 1988.
92. *Medicinskaja Gazeta*, 2 September 1987, number 70 (4723) p3.
93. A. M. Brandt, *American Journal of Public Health*, volume 78, number 4, p370.
94. *Le Point*, Paris, 15 February 1988.
95. as reference 94.
96. Information from Elections Division, Secretary of State, State of California, June 1988.
97. *Daily Telegraph*, London, 6 March 1987.
98. W. F. Buckley, writing in *International Herald Tribune*, 19 March 1986.
99. P.D. Cleary et al, *Journal of the American Medical Association*, 2 October 1987, volume 258, pp1,757-62.
100. Information from Dr Lutz Gürtler, July 1988.
101 *New York Times*, 16 April 1988.
102. Office of Assistant Secretary of Defense for Health Affairs, Washington DC, July 1988.
103. Information from David FitzSimons, Bureau of Hygiene and Tropical Diseases, London, June 1988.
104. Dr Halfdan Mahler, opening address, World Summit of Health Ministers on programmes for AIDS prevention, London, January 1988.
105. Dr J. M. Mann, address to the World Summit of Health Ministers on programmes for AIDS prevention, London, January 1988.
106. G. Friedland, *Journal of the American Medical Association*, 20 May 1988, volume 259, number 19, pp2,898-9. Emphasis as in the original.
107. *Chairman's Draft Recommendations for the Final Report*, Presidential Commission on the Human Immunodeficiency Virus Epidemic, Washington DC, June 1988, p194.
108. *Confronting AIDS: Update 1988*, Institute of Medicine of the National Academy of Sciences, Washington DC, June 1988, Chapter 4, p4. Emphasis as in the original.
109. as reference 106.

Index

BLAMING OTHERS

Prejudice, race and worldwide AIDS

by Renée Sabatier
and Tade Aina, Patricia Ardila, Erlinda Bolido,
Philippe Engelhard, K.S. Jayaraman, Dave Moyo,
Dorothy Kweyu Munyakho, Hikloch Ogola, Seun
Ogunseitan, Abib Samb, Moussa Seck, Lazaro Timmo.

WORLDAIDS

By late 1988 Panos hopes to be publishing a new regular inter-disciplinary newsletter called *WORLDAIDS.* Produced in collaboration with the London Bureau of Hygiene and Tropical Diseases this publication will be a compre-hensive overview of AIDS emphasising the effect on the Third World. If you would be interested in finding out more about how to get *WORLDAIDS* please tick the order form below and you will be sent the relevant information as soon as it is available.

The global spread of AIDS is triggering dangerous epidemics of blame and racial prejudice. AIDS is being blamed on gays, or on drug addicts, or on blacks. Britain has blamed African students, the USA has blamed Haitians, Africa has blamed Europeans, Japan has blamed foreigners, the French right has blamed Arab immigrants.

With contributions from 12 Third World journalists and researchers, *Blaming Others* by Renée Sabatier analyses some of the most loaded, emotive and confusing issues connected with AIDS. Is blame undermining AIDS prevention? Where did the virus come from — and does it matter? How widespread is "promiscuity", what is the role of prostitution, is the spread of AIDS linked to other sexual diseases? Has Western reporting on AIDS in the Third World been hysterical? Is AIDS research racially biased? Are some ethnic groups especially vulnerable to AIDS? Should governments screen foreign students?

Blaming Others argues that the AIDS virus is a misery-seeking missile, increasingly selecting its targets from among the world's most disadvantaged communities: black and Latino minorities in the United States, and Third World countries in Africa and the Caribbean.

These communities are doubly vulnerable: from social and economic deprivation, and from a deadly lack of AIDS information. The result? A US white diagnosed with AIDS is likely to survive two years; a US black only 19 weeks, says *Blaming Others.* And of the world's 20 most severe national AIDS epidemics, all but two are in developing countries.

Blaming Others is the first international analysis of the AIDS epidemic of blame. It argues that, in every country and on every level from the local to the global, blame and prejudice are undermining AIDS campaigns.

For ordering information contact:

New Society Publishers/West   or   **The Panos Institute**
PO Box 582   1409 King Street
Santa Cruz, CA 95061   Alexandria, VA 22314